Addicted
to *Failure*

Why the Rehab System Doesn't Work and What Must Change

JIMMIE APPLEGATE

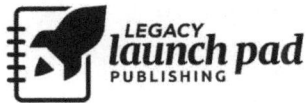

LEGACY
launch pad
PUBLISHING

ISBN: 978-1-968339-88-3 (ebook)

ISBN: 978-1-968339-87-6 (paperback)

Disclaimer

This book represents the author's personal opinions, experiences and interpretations of publicly available information and professional practices within the addiction treatment field. It is not intended to make factual allegations about any specific organization, facility or individual.

All references to treatment centers, professionals, institutions and programs are presented for discussion and illustrative purposes only. Where real entities are mentioned, the information reflects the author's good faith understanding at the time of writing based on publicly available sources, and no implication of misconduct, malpractice or wrongdoing is intended or should be inferred.

Certain names, identifying details and circumstances have been changed, combined or fictionalized to protect privacy. Any resemblance to actual persons, living or deceased, or to actual organizations or events is purely coincidental.

The content of this book is for informational and educational purposes only. It does not constitute medical, psychological or legal advice, and should not be relied upon as a substitute for consultation with qualified professionals. The author and publisher disclaim any liability for actions taken or not taken based on the contents of this work.

The views expressed are solely those of the author and do not necessarily represent those of any organization or professional association with which the author is or has been affiliated.

For more information about Jimmie Applegate and his work, scan the QR code below:

To Jason, for lighting the fire, thx Bro.

Contents

Preface

I wish this book didn't need to exist. I wish the stories that fill detox centers, emergency rooms and back alleys, stories of human suffering recycled through a system that is supposed to heal but too often only manages to manage, were only fiction.

But here we are.

The addiction recovery industry is broken. Not cracked. Not merely outdated. *Broken.* And it is costing us lives.

I write from experience, both as a patient and as a professional. My personal journey through addiction recovery involved multiple relapses and extensive exploration of treatment modalities. As someone who experienced repeated treatment episodes, I understand the challenges faced by individuals who do not achieve sustained recovery through traditional approaches. My sobriety began within the 12-step program, but this single modality proved insufficient for maintaining long-term sobriety.

Through dedicated study of recovery methodologies, I developed a comprehensive toolkit incorporating multiple evidence-based approaches. My experience demonstrated that sustainable recovery often requires a personalized combination of interventions rather than reliance on any single treatment philosophy, a discovery I made largely through independent exploration rather than systematic clinical guidance.

While initially frustrating to observe others achieving stable recovery more rapidly, I now understand that my extended journey provided invaluable insights into addiction's complexity and the limitations of one-size-fits-all treatment approaches. This experience drives my commitment to ensuring others do not have to navigate recovery through trial and error when comprehensive, individualized treatment should be available from the outset.

This now informs my professional path forward—I aim to change the way recovery is done. I aim to make a greater difference in the lives of those who seek lasting change.

For decades, we've trusted a system built on models that haven't evolved meaningfully since the mid-20th century. We've clung to programs that treat addiction as a moral failing or spiritual void, with science left waiting outside the door. We've accepted revolving-door rehabs, 30-day miracles and insurance-driven discharge dates. We've mistaken profit for progress.

Meanwhile, overdose deaths have skyrocketed. Entire communities have been hollowed out. Families bury their loved ones while treatment conglomerate CEOs cash checks and pharmaceutical executives dodge accountability.

What you're about to read is not a comfortable book. It's a confrontation. It's a reckoning.

This book rips apart the polished brochures and exposes what's really going on behind the locked doors of detox centers and luxury rehabs. It dissects how the business of addiction treatment feeds on the very suffering it claims to heal. It throws darts at sacred cows, including the 12-step model, and demands a new way forward grounded in neuroscience, trauma-informed care and actual healing.

This book isn't just critique. It's a blueprint.

Each chapter dissects what's broken: the antiquated treatment models peddled as innovation, the financial machinery that profits from relapse, the gaping wounds where science should be. But it doesn't stop at diagnosis. It offers a radical reimagining of what recovery could be—what it *must* be—if we're serious about saving lives instead of just managing symptoms. It spends time with fellow addicts, people who have been through (and are still trying to navigate) an increasingly fraught, complicated system, whose stories I'm honored to tell.

It dares to ask: *What if we didn't just help people survive addiction, but actually helped them transform their lives?* What if treatment wasn't just about removing substances but about restoring purpose, connection and genuine healing? What if we built a system that worked for the many, not just the privileged few?

If you've been through this system, shuttled between detoxes, handed platitudes instead of tools, blamed for the failure of methods that were designed to fail, you already know the truth in your bones. If you're working in this system, fighting against protocols you know are inadequate, you probably do too—and maybe you're exhausted from the moral injury of participating in something that falls so short of what could be. If you're watching someone you love drown while supposedly being "treated," maybe you're wondering why real hope always seems just out of reach, while expensive false promises are everywhere.

This book is for you. And for everyone who's had enough of watching people die while we keep doing the same damn thing, enough of calling failure "the nature of the disease," enough of a system that measures success by insurance payouts rather than transformed lives.

Let's tear it down—not just the buildings and programs, but the outdated thinking, the profit-driven models and the comfortable lies that keep us stuck.

Let's build something that works, something grounded in neuroscience and compassion, something that honors both evidence and lived experience, something worthy of the human potential for healing that we witness every day despite the system, not because of it.

The revolution in addiction treatment isn't coming. It's here. In these pages. In your hands.

And it starts now.

For too long, I've wrestled with insurance companies that prioritize profit over people, watching them deny coverage for innovative treatments while funding the same failed approaches. I'm tired of waiting for bureaucrats to approve what we already know works. I'm done with a system that measures success by quarterly reports rather than transformed lives.

That's why I'm not waiting anymore. It's time to go around them, through them, over them to create new pathways for funding real recovery. There are people out there who share this vision, who believe in supporting evidence-based treatment regardless of what some insurance executive decides is "cost-effective." If you're one of them, if you're tired of watching the system fail the people you care about, I invite you to join this movement.

Visit BeaconCharities.com or download the 10foraddiction app to discover how we're building a new way forward. Together, we can create a system that actually serves those seeking recovery instead of the corporations profiting from their suffering.

Broken at the Foundation: Conflicting Addiction Models and Their Consequences

The idea that there's a single program that works for everyone with addiction is like saying there's one treatment for all forms of cancer. It's not just wrong; it's harmful, because it prevents people from finding approaches that might actually work for them.

The Square Peg: Why One Size Never Fits All

Alex stared at the laminated 12-step poster on the church basement wall. This was his fourth meeting this week, his third different group and his seventh attempt at working the program over the past five years. Around him, heads nodded as a speaker described his "moment of surrender" and how turning his will over to a Higher Power had saved him.

"I was exactly where you are," the speaker said, making eye contact with Alex. "Fighting the program. Thinking I was different. Special. But once I admitted I was powerless and really worked the steps, everything changed."

Alex shifted uncomfortably. He wasn't fighting anything. He'd read the Big Book cover to cover, twice. He'd found a sponsor, worked the steps, shared in meetings. He'd surrendered so many times he'd lost count. Yet here he was again, 30 days sober and feeling like an impostor.

Outside after the meeting, his sponsor Mike clapped a hand on his shoulder. "You're thinking too much again," he said. "Your best thinking got you here, remember? You need to let go and let God."

Alex nodded, but something inside him recoiled. The constant focus on character defects made his already crushing shame worse. The Higher Power concept felt forced. And the disease model didn't capture his experience of using substances to numb the hypervigilance from childhood trauma.

"I'll try harder," Alex said, the words hollow in his mouth.

That night, he pulled out his recovery journal. Six separate attempts at the program, each ending the same way—with him feeling more broken, more hopeless. The common denominator was him, wasn't it? His failure. His inadequacy.

His therapist had suggested last week that maybe the problem wasn't him.

"The 12-step approach works wonderfully for some people," she'd said. "But it's not the only path to recovery. Your brain chemistry, your trauma history, your personality type all affect how you respond to different recovery models."

The idea that there could be a different approach felt both liberating and terrifying. In every meeting, they reinforced that this program was the only thing that worked.

He opened his laptop and typed: "alternatives to 12-step recovery." The search results surprised him—SMART Recovery, Refuge Recovery, LifeRing, trauma-focused approaches.

The next morning, Alex woke up to a text from Mike: "Missed you at the 6 am meeting. Remember, meeting makers make it."

The familiar guilt rose up, but then something shifted. Maybe he wasn't failing the program. Maybe the program was failing him.

He texted back: "Taking a different path for a while. Thank you for everything."

As he walked into his first SMART Recovery meeting, a woman greeted him with a smile. "First time?"

Alex nodded.

"Welcome," she said. "The only requirement here is a desire to work on your recovery. How that looks is up to you."

Something loosened in Alex's chest—a knot of shame he'd carried for so long he'd forgotten it was there. He wasn't broken. He was just different. And maybe that was okay.

The Fundamental Disagreement: What Really Causes Addiction?

Alex's story highlights a critical reality in addiction treatment: Experts fundamentally disagree about what addiction actually is and what causes it. This disagreement isn't merely academic; it shapes every aspect of how we approach recovery, from the language we use to the treatments we offer to the expectations we place on those struggling with substance use.

The numbers don't lie. Despite decades of research, billions in funding and an entire industry dedicated to addiction treatment, success rates hover below a dismal 40%.[1] For a medical intervention, that's not just disappointing—it's a crisis.

Here's the uncomfortable truth: Most addiction treatment programs are stuck in an outdated paradigm. They're addressing symptoms while missing the underlying transformation that makes recovery possible. And they're doing so because they're built on fundamentally conflicting models of what addiction is in the first place.

The modern battlefield of addiction science is littered with competing theories, each claiming superior understanding of what drives addictive behavior and how to address it. These models don't just disagree; they often directly contradict each other.

View #1

For trauma-informed practitioners like Dr. Gabor Maté, addiction isn't primarily about substances; it's about emotional wounds seeking relief. **"A hurt is at the center of all addictive behaviors,"** he explains in his 2008 book *In the Realm of Hungry Ghosts: Close Encounters with Addiction.*[2] "The wound may not be as deep and the ache not as excruciating, and it may even be entirely hidden—but it's there."

Research increasingly supports this perspective. The landmark Adverse Childhood Experiences (ACE) study, originally conducted at Kaiser Permanente in the mid-1990s, found that people with four or more adverse childhood experiences were 10 times more likely to develop substance addiction than those with none. Studies of treatment populations consistently find trauma rates of 60 to 90% among people seeking addiction treatment.[3]

Trauma creates neurobiological changes that prime the brain for addiction. It dysregulates the stress response system, alters the brain's reward pathways and impairs the prefrontal cortex—the same systems affected by addictive substances. In many cases, substance use begins as an attempt to self-medicate the unbearable symptoms of unresolved trauma.

Yet this trauma-informed perspective is just one of several competing models.

View #2

The National Institute on Drug Abuse (NIDA), led by Dr. Nora Volkow, champions a very different view, commonly known as the **"brain disease model."** This approach describes addiction as "a chronic, relapsing brain disorder characterized by compulsive drug seeking and use despite adverse consequences."[4]

This model suggests that addiction changes the brain's reward system, stress systems and executive function in fundamental ways that make it increasingly difficult for the person to control their substance use.

According to this model, repeated substance use causes measurable changes in brain structure and function, particularly in regions governing reward, motivation, learning, judgment and memory. These changes explain why people continue using substances despite negative consequences—their brains have been altered in ways that make stopping extremely difficult.

The disease model has gained substantial traction in medical and scientific communities. It's backed by impressive neuroimaging studies showing physical changes in the brains of people with addictions. It offers a clear explanation for why quitting is so difficult, and it reduces stigma by framing addiction as a medical condition rather than a moral failing.

View #3

But critics argue that the brain disease model misinterprets the evidence. Dr. Marc Lewis, neuroscientist and author of *The Biology of Desire: Why Addiction Is Not a Disease*, offers a third perspective that challenges both the trauma model and the disease model while incorporating elements of each.[5]

Addiction is a developmental process, not a disease, according to proponents of this model, who see addiction as a form of accelerated learning wherein the brain does exactly what it's designed to do: form strong habits around experiences that provide relief or pleasure. The brain changes associated with addiction are not evidence of pathology, but rather of the brain's extraordinary capacity to learn and adapt.

From this developmental perspective, addiction isn't a

disease to be treated or cured but a powerful habit to be unlearned and replaced. It acknowledges the neurobiological components of addiction while rejecting the notion that these changes represent a permanent pathology.

View #4

A fourth perspective comes from Dr. Patrick Carnes, pioneer in sexual addiction treatment and founder of the International Institute for Trauma and Addiction Professionals (IITAP). Dr. Carnes emphasizes addiction as fundamentally a disorder of intimacy, explaining that early attachment experiences create templates for how we connect with others. When these are disrupted, the theory goes, addiction can become a substitute for healthy connection.

Dr. Carnes' research with over 4,400 sex addicts found that only 8% tested as having secure attachment, compared to roughly 60% in the general population.[6] His attachment-based model extends beyond sexual addiction to substance use, viewing addictive behaviors as maladaptive attempts to regulate the attachment system, the fundamental human need for connection and safety.

This perspective aligns with mounting research showing consistent associations between insecure attachment and substance use disorders. A meta-analysis of 34 prospective studies involving over 56,000 participants found significant associations between insecure attachment and later substance use problems, with the relationship persisting across different types of substances.[7]

Dr. Philip Flores, clinical psychologist and author of *Addiction as an Attachment Disorder*, reinforces this perspective, arguing that "individuals who become dependent on addictive substances cannot regulate their emotions, self-care, self-esteem, and relationships" due to early attachment disruptions.[8] As Johann Hari famously observed, "The opposite of addiction isn't sobriety—it's connection."[9]

Research by Dr. Andreas Schindler at the University Medical Center Hamburg-Eppendorf demonstrates that substance abuse can be understood as "self-medication," or an attempt to compensate for lacking attachment strategies. His studies show different attachment patterns predict different types of substance use: Heroin users predominantly show fearful-avoidant attachment, while cannabis users display more dismissing-avoidant patterns.[10]

The attachment disorder model suggests that addiction fills the void left by disrupted early relationships, with substances providing the regulation, comfort and predictability that secure attachments normally offer. This framework explains why traditional approaches focused solely on removing substances often fail—they address the symptom while leaving the underlying attachment wounds untreated.

View #5

These scientific perspectives stand in stark contrast to the traditional 12-step view that has dominated treatment centers across America for decades: the view that addiction is primarily a spiritual disease requiring spiritual solutions.

As one 12-step text states: "We were spiritually sick. As we became subjects of King Alcohol, shivering denizens of his mad realm, the chilling vapor that is loneliness settled down." [11] The solution, according to this model, is not trauma resolution or neurobiological intervention, but spiritual awakening, surrendering to a Higher Power, making amends for past wrongs and helping others with the same condition.

These competing models don't just disagree on details; they fundamentally contradict each other on what addiction is and how it should be addressed:

- Is addiction a brain disease requiring medical intervention, or is the disease model itself a misinterpretation of the evidence?
- Is addiction primarily a response to trauma, or can it develop in the absence of significant psychological wounds?
- Is recovery about managing a chronic condition, healing emotional pain, rewiring neural pathways or spiritual transformation?

These aren't merely academic questions. They shape every aspect of how we approach addiction, from insurance coverage to treatment protocols to the language we use with those seeking help.

When someone enters treatment, they're not just receiving care—they're being indoctrinated into a particular model of understanding their condition. If that model doesn't match their experience, they're often told they're in denial, resistant or not ready for recovery, rather than the system recognizing that the model itself might be inadequate for their situation. Put differently: If addiction is primarily spiritual, then prayer, moral inventory and surrender to a Higher Power are the logical solutions; if it's primarily a brain disease, then medication and neurobiological interventions take precedence; if it's a response to trauma, then trauma therapy becomes essential; if addiction is a learning disorder, then new learning and development are key to lifelong recovery; if it's an attachment disorder, then relationship healing takes center stage.

A person may not have all these ailments, but it's probable that they have a combination of a few of them. If the recovery center that they're attending doesn't see it that way, they will not get the help they need for lifelong recovery.

For someone like Alex, caught in this crossfire of competing theories, the consequences are deeply personal. His inability to find healing through the spiritual approach wasn't evidence of personal failure; it reflected the mismatch between the treatment model and his actual condition. Yet the system's response was to double down on the same approach, deepening his shame rather than reconsidering the treatment paradigm.

Each of these perspectives—trauma-informed, disease model, developmental learning, spiritual and attachment disorder—represents legitimate expertise from thoughtful professionals offering evidence-based solutions. These are brilliant minds tackling an extraordinarily complex problem, and there's validity in every approach presented here. The challenge isn't that any of these viewpoints are wrong, it's that they're not encountered by those seeking help.

When someone struggling with addiction searches for answers, or when a well-intentioned treatment center seeks the best approach for their patients, these models are often presented as competing truths rather than complementary insights. A person seeking recovery may encounter the disease model at one facility, trauma-informed care at another and spiritual solutions at a third, with each approach claiming to hold the key to lasting recovery. This fragmentation can lead to confusion about their own particular challenge, leaving both individuals and treatment providers unsure which path to pursue.

The goal isn't to declare one perspective superior, but to help seekers understand these different lenses so they can make informed decisions about their recovery journey. Each model offers valuable tools for different individuals facing different circumstances, so the question isn't which one is right, but which combination might work best for each person's unique situation.

When practitioners can't even agree on what the problem is, how can they possibly develop effective solutions for the millions of people whose lives hang in the balance?

The Religion of Recovery: When Spiritual Solutions Fall Short

It's a controversial reality in addiction treatment: The dominance of a spiritual approach fails most people who try it.

Alcoholics Anonymous and its many offshoots represent the most widely recognized approach to addiction recovery in America. Founded in 1935 by two desperate alcoholics—a New York stockbroker and an Ohio surgeon—AA has morphed into an empire of recovery that spans the globe. The 12 Steps have been adapted for everything from narcotics to gambling, sex addiction to overeating. They've been integrated into residential treatment centers, outpatient programs and court-mandated rehabilitation. [12]

This wasn't the result of scientific validation or comparative effectiveness research. It was an accident of history, timing and cultural resonance.

The 12-step approach emerged during a particular historical moment when medical and psychological treatments for addiction were limited, Dr. Lance Dodes explains in his 2014 book *The Sober Truth: Debunking the Bad Science Behind 12-Step Programs and the Rehab Industry.* The program filled a vacuum and became entrenched before scientific methods could evaluate its effectiveness.[13]

The monopolization of addiction treatment happened through three key mechanisms:

1. The absence of alternatives. When AA emerged in the 1930s, medical approaches to addiction were primitive and often harmful. Psychological treatments were in their infancy. The 12 Steps offered structure, community and hope when little else existed.

2. Religious and cultural alignment. AA's spiritual foundation resonated with America's predominantly Christian culture. Its emphasis on character, moral inventory and redemption aligned with prevailing values. Government and religious institutions embraced and promoted it.
3. The recovery industry's economic incentives. As residential treatment centers proliferated in the 1980s and 1990s, they adopted the 12-step model because it was free, familiar and didn't require specialized training to implement. Insurance companies found it convenient to fund a standardized approach with a built-in aftercare system that cost them nothing.[14]

The result? A recovery monoculture where one approach, developed by nonprofessionals nearly a century ago, became the default intervention for a complex brain condition affecting millions of diverse individuals.

This wouldn't be problematic if the approach worked universally. But it doesn't.

Dr. Dodes' review of the research found that "the actual success rate of AA, for those who attend at least one meeting, is approximately 5-10%," a far cry from the near-universal effectiveness claimed by some 12-step advocates.[15]

The Cochrane Collaboration, an independent research organization known for its rigorous systematic reviews, concluded in 2020 that "there is high quality evidence that [12-step facilitation approaches] are as effective as other established treatments."[16] Note the phrasing: "as effective as other established treatments"—not more effective, and certainly not universally effective.

This research suggests that 12-step programs work about as well as other approaches, helping some people and not others.

The factors that predict success in 12-step programs are reveal-ing. Research shows that individuals who already have religious or spiritual beliefs, who are comfortable with group settings, who resonate with concepts like powerlessness and character defects and who have strong social support are more likely to benefit.

Conversely, those with trauma histories, those who are atheist or agnostic, those with co-occurring mental health conditions and those who struggle with the concept of power-lessness often fare poorly in 12-step programs.

For these individuals, the emphasis on spiritual solutions doesn't address the underlying drivers of their addiction. The focus on powerlessness may reinforce feelings of helplessness rather than empowerment. The moral inventory may intensify shame rather than healing it. And the one-day-at-a-time approach may provide structure, but not the skills needed for long-term recovery.

As Dr. Lewis notes, "Addicts need empowerment and self-direction in order to change. But the medicalization of addic-tion turns them into patients: obedient, passive, and power-less."[17]

Before moving forward, let me be clear: I'm not categori-cally opposed to 12-step programs. I achieved my own sobriety through a 12-step program, and I've witnessed count-less lives transformed by this approach. My issue isn't with the programs themselves; it's how they're sold: how they're posi-tioned as the one-stop shop, the fix-all, The One and Only Solution. This becomes problematic when we consider the Cochrane research findings—12-step approaches aren't more effective than other evidence-based treatments, and they're certainly not universally effective. Herein lies the problem. If it's not universally effective, why is it that everyone in the universe is recommending it?

Think about this with me. If you were to disclose to your primary care physician that you think you have an addiction, they are going to tell you to go to a 12-step meeting.

Discuss this topic with your psychologist, psychiatrist, social worker or counselor? Easy: Go to a 12-step meeting.

Get in trouble with the law because of alcohol or illicit substances and wind up in the drunk tank overnight; what's the cop going to say to you? Go to a 12-step meeting.

Your lawyer, legal counsel, judge and probation officer: 12-step meeting.

Dare to speak with your cousin, mom, uncle, any family member or your best friend's dad?

How about your local clergy? I dare you: Ask a bishop, priest, father, pastor. 12-step meeting.

I could go on, but what's the *real* point?

It's this: These recommendations come from a place of genuine care—people want to help and believe they're steering someone toward recovery. The problem is that a 12-step meeting has become the only path most people know to recommend, not because it's the only effective approach, but because it's the only approach they're aware of. 12-step programs, while valuable for many, aren't the universal solution, and there's a significant likelihood that someone seeking help may need a different approach entirely, or at minimum, additional interventions beyond 12-step meetings. I'm going to say this one more time: People, especially professional people who are dishing out advice, need to be informed that the 12-step meeting is *not* the one-stop shop, and that there is a good chance that the friend they are advising needs a solution *other than* or *in addition to* a 12-step meeting.

The Collateral Damage: Real Lives Caught in the Crossfire

While experts battle over models and theories, real people pay the price.

Alex's story is far from unique. Millions of individuals seeking recovery find themselves trapped in treatment approaches that don't match their needs, not because these approaches are universally ineffective, but because they're being applied universally despite evidence that they work selectively.

The battle between competing addiction models creates a fractured foundation for the entire field of addiction treatment. Without consensus on the fundamental nature of the problem, we've built treatment systems that often work at cross-purposes, leaving those seeking help caught in the crossfire of competing theories.

The addiction field's inability to reach consensus on these fundamental questions creates a treatment landscape where what help you receive depends more on which door you happen to walk through than on your specific needs. A person entering a 12-step-based facility will be treated for a spiritual malady, while the same person entering a medication-first program will be treated for a brain disease—with radically different approaches and outcomes.

The consequences are severe:

- People with trauma histories are told their addiction is a disease requiring medication and abstinence, with little attention to the emotional wounds driving their substance use.
- Those who don't respond to spiritual approaches are labeled as "constitutionally incapable of being honest with themselves" rather than recognized as needing a different model.[18]
- Individuals with co-occurring mental health conditions are told to focus exclusively on their addiction, often being advised to stop psychiatric medications that may be essential for their stability.
- Those who question the disease model are told they're in denial about their condition, while those who reject spiritual solutions are warned

they're doomed to "jails, institutions or death."
[19]

This one-size-fits-all approach creates what Dr. Dodes calls a "false consensus effect," which is the assumption that most people share your beliefs and experiences. When someone fails to connect with the dominant approach, they're told they're "not working the program correctly" or "haven't hit bottom yet." The possibility that the program itself might be mismatched to their needs is rarely considered.

The human cost is staggering. People cycle through multiple treatment episodes, each reinforcing the idea that they, not the treatment approach, are the problem. Each "failure" deepens shame and hopelessness, making it increasingly difficult to sustain the motivation needed for lasting change.

The irony is that we now have multiple evidence-based approaches to addiction treatment, each effective for different populations:

- Cognitive behavioral therapy (CBT) shows strong results for many substance use disorders, particularly when combined with motivational approaches.
- Medication-assisted treatment (MAT) significantly reduces mortality for opioid use disorders when implemented properly.
- Trauma-focused therapies like EMDR and Seeking Safety show promise for those with co-occurring trauma and addiction.
- Mindfulness-based approaches like mindfulness-based relapse prevention demonstrate effectiveness for preventing relapse.
- Other options include the community reinforcement approach, dialectical behavior therapy and acceptance and commitment therapy.

The list of evidence-based treatments continues
to grow.

Yet many people never encounter these alternatives
because they're trapped in a treatment system dominated by a
single paradigm—one that may not match their needs at all.

The consequences extend beyond individual suffering.
The societal cost of our fractured approach to addiction is
measured in lives lost, families destroyed and billions of
dollars wasted on ineffective interventions.

The opioid crisis alone claims over 100,000 American lives
annually, many of whom had previously sought treatment but
didn't find approaches that worked for them.[20] How many
might have been saved if they'd been offered interventions
matched to their specific needs rather than forced into a one-
size-fits-all model?

The solution isn't abandoning any particular model, but
recognizing that multiple models are needed to address the
complex and varied nature of addiction. Different individuals
require different approaches based on their unique circumstances: their trauma history, brain chemistry, psychological
makeup, social context and personal values.

As we move forward, we must build a treatment system
that embraces this diversity of approaches rather than clinging
to a single dominant paradigm. We need a system that asks
not "Is this the right model?" but "Is this the right model for
this particular person?"

Alex found his path eventually, but not without years of
unnecessary suffering, shame and self-doubt. How many
others are still lost in the crossfire of competing addiction
theories, unable to find approaches that match their needs?

The foundation of addiction treatment is broken, fractured by conflicting models and theories that too often prioritize ideological purity over practical effectiveness. Until we

address this fundamental problem, we'll continue to fail the millions of individuals and families affected by addiction.

But there is hope. By understanding these competing models—their strengths, limitations and the evidence behind them—we can begin to build a "Customized" approach to addiction treatment. One that recognizes the validity of multiple perspectives while prioritizing the needs of the individual seeking help over the theoretical purity of any particular model.

In the chapters that follow, we'll explore specific failures of the current system and how they stem from this fractured foundation. More importantly, we'll examine how a new, "Customized" approach can transform addiction treatment from a revolving door of failure to a pathway toward lasting healing and growth.

2

The Business of Failure: Financial Exploitation and Outdated Models

Addiction is a chronic condition, and treating it with short-term interventions alone is akin to treating someone with diabetes by giving them a week's worth of insulin.

The 30-Day Fallacy: Built for Billing, Not for Healing

Nathan sat in the office of the treatment center's admissions coordinator, a thick folder of medical records heavy on his lap. This was his fourth rehab in three years—the third one this year alone.

"So, Nathan," the coordinator said, peering at him over tortoiseshell glasses, "tell me what brings you back to treatment."

He took a deep breath, feeling the familiar mix of hope and exhaustion. "I relapsed," he said quietly. "Again."

The coordinator nodded sympathetically, tapping notes into her computer. "And how long were you sober after your last treatment?"

Nathan stared at the wall behind her, at the framed certificates and stock photos of mountains meant to inspire hope. "Forty-three days."

"That's actually quite good," she said, offering a gentle smile. "Many people don't make it that long."

He managed a weak smile in return, though inside he wondered if that was supposed to be comforting. "Thank you. I mean, I tried. I really did try."

"I can see that," she said warmly. "Your insurance should cover another 28-day stay. We'll need pre-authorization, of course."

"Twenty-eight days," Nathan repeated, his voice thoughtful rather than accusatory. "Just like last time."

"Well, yes. That's the standard program length that most insurance companies approve."

Nathan shifted in his chair, choosing his words carefully. "I appreciate everything you all do here, I really do. But I'm wondering...do you think 28 days might not be enough time? I mean, I completed the program successfully last time. And the time before. But something isn't quite clicking for the long-term."

The coordinator's expression remained patient but guarded. "Every recovery journey is different, Nathan. Perhaps this time the program will resonate differently—"

"I hope so," he said earnestly. "I really hope so. It's just..." He paused, running his hand through his hair. "I keep thinking about how long it took me to get sick, you know? Years of using. And I'm trying to understand how four weeks can undo all that damage."

She nodded understandingly. "We do offer extended care options. Another 30, 60 or 90 days in our residential program. Of course, insurance rarely covers that, so it would be out of pocket."

"How much would something like that cost?" Nathan asked, though he already suspected the answer.

"For the extended residential program? About $30,000 per month."

Nathan's shoulders sagged slightly. "I see. So my options

are the 28 days my insurance covers, or..." He trailed off, doing the mental math. "I want to get better. I really do. But I've already spent over $15,000 in copays and deductibles on treatment, and my family has been so supportive financially, but we're just not in a position to..."

The coordinator's expression softened. "I understand completely. Insurance limitations are one of the biggest challenges we face in this field."

Nathan looked up hopefully. "Is there any research on whether longer treatment works better? I'm not questioning your program—it's good, really good. I'm just trying to understand why I keep ending up back here despite doing everything I was taught."

"That's a very thoughtful question," she replied carefully. "The research does suggest that longer treatment episodes tend to have better outcomes. But our hands are somewhat tied by what insurance will authorize."

Nathan nodded slowly, absorbing this. "I guess what I'm struggling with is that each time I leave, I feel hopeful and prepared. But then around week six or seven, something shifts. It's like my brain isn't quite ready yet, you know? And I wonder if maybe it needs more time to heal."

He stood, gathering his folder with renewed determination. "But I'm grateful you have a program at all. And I'm going to give it everything I have this time too."

At the door, he turned back. "I'll be here tomorrow for intake. Because even if 28 days isn't perfect, it's still something. And maybe this time will be different."

The coordinator watched him go, something sad and knowing in her eyes.

Selling Hope, Delivering Relapse: The Economics of Treatment Failure

The addiction treatment industry has mastered a perfect

business model: sell an ineffective product, blame the customer when it fails, then welcome them back with open arms to try again. It was a $16.22 billion market in 2024 and is projected to reach $36.83 billion by 2034, with a growth rate of over 10% annually.[21] This explosive growth isn't driven by breakthrough treatment innovations; it's fueled by repeated admissions of the same patients cycling through the system.

Unlike other healthcare sectors where success is measured by patient outcomes, the addiction treatment industry profits directly from failure. When a treatment program doesn't produce lasting recovery, clients return for another round of expensive care. And another. And another.

The numbers are stark: Within one year following treatment, relapse rates range from 40 to 60%.[22] Some studies suggest that only 5 to 10% of people who attend 12-step programs achieve lasting sobriety.[23] For residential treatment programs, estimates vary, but studies indicate that between 40 and 80% of patients relapse within a year of discharge.[24]

Yet this abysmal track record hasn't hurt the industry's bottom line. Quite the opposite: It's created a revolving door that keeps treatment centers' beds filled and their revenue streams flowing. A single 30-day inpatient stay can cost anywhere from $5,000 to $97,000, with the average hovering around $12,500. Luxury facilities charge upward of $50,000 to $100,000 per month.[25]

The system isn't designed to cure addiction; it's designed to keep people cycling through it. If rehab actually worked long-term, these centers would lose their most reliable source of income—repeat clients.

Let's do some easy math with the averages: If a treatment center charges $12,500 for a 30-day program, and 60% of their clients return for at least one more stay, that's an additional $7,500 in revenue per initial client—just from expected failure. For a facility with 60 beds turning over monthly, that's potentially $450,000 in additional annual revenue generated solely by treatment failure. I'm going to invite you to pause here for a moment: to reread this paragraph and just let that sink in.

What other business could survive, let alone thrive, with a 60% failure rate? Imagine if 60% of cars broke down within months of purchase, or if 60% of surgeries required immediate revision. In those industries, such failure would trigger recalls, lawsuits and regulatory crackdowns. In addiction treatment, it's simply accepted as the norm.

More troubling still is how this business model shifts blame onto patients. When someone relapses after treatment, they're rarely told "Our program failed to give you adequate tools for lasting recovery." Instead, they hear "You weren't ready," "You didn't work the program hard enough" or "You need to surrender more."

This systematic blame-shifting serves a crucial business function: It protects the industry's reputation while ensuring clients return with their wallets open and their self-esteem in tatters, a perfect setup for another expensive round of "treatment" that statistically has little chance of producing lasting change.

The sad truth is that most treatment centers know their programs aren't long enough or comprehensive enough to create lasting neurological change. The brain needs months, not weeks, to heal from addiction. But rather than challenging the insurance-dictated 28-day model or investing in research for more effective approaches, many facilities have simply adapted their business plans to profit from the revolving door.

The Accidental Monopoly: How 12 Step Cornered the Market

As residential treatment centers proliferated in the 1980s

and 1990s, they discovered that the 12-step model offered a perfect solution to their business challenges. It was free, requiring no licensing fees or specialized staff training. It provided built-in aftercare through community meetings, allowing facilities to claim "continuing care" without cost. When patients relapsed, responsibility shifted to the individual's failure to "work the program" rather than the treatment method itself. And as a spiritual program, it required no scientific validation, avoiding the costly burden of evidence-based practice.

The result? A treatment landscape where, in my experience, approximately 70 to 80% of residential programs in America are self-proclaimed "12-step-centric," despite mounting evidence that 12 Step works effectively for only a minority of patients. This is down from reports in the '80s and '90s, which showed 80 to 95% of the centers were built around the 12-step model. As I mentioned earlier, the Cochrane Collaboration concluded in 2020 that "there is high quality evidence that [12-step facilitation approaches] are as effective as other established treatments."[26] Remember: "*as effective as other established treatments*," not *more* effective, and certainly not universally effective.

Yet the monopoly persists, leaving those who don't respond to the 12-step approach—often the majority—trapped in a cycle of treatment, failure, shame and relapse.

This economic entrenchment has created an unusual situation where evidence-based alternatives struggle to gain market share despite superior outcomes for many populations. Cognitive behavioral therapy, motivational enhancement therapy and trauma-informed approaches often show better results than 12-step programs, but they require specialized training, ongoing supervision and individualized treatment planning, all of which cost money.

The financial incentives are clear: Why invest in expensive, evidence-based treatments when you can offer a free, widely accepted alternative that shifts the blame for failure onto the patient? This economic logic has trapped the industry in a treatment approach developed nearly a century ago, leaving millions of people without access to interventions that might actually work for their specific needs and circumstances.

Big Pharma's Double Dip: Creating Addicts, Then "Treating" Them

In 1996, Purdue Pharma introduced OxyContin with an aggressive marketing campaign unlike anything the pharmaceutical industry had seen before. The company spent millions convincing doctors that this powerful opioid, which is chemically similar to heroin, posed minimal addiction risk when used for pain management. Sales representatives received bonuses exceeding $70 million for pushing the drug, while the company's internal documents revealed they knew about its addiction potential from the start.[27]

The results were catastrophic. Prescriptions for opioids skyrocketed from about 76 million in 1991 to nearly 219 million by 2011. Addiction rates surged in parallel, creating what would become known as the opioid epidemic, a crisis that has claimed over 500,000 American lives through overdose since 1999.[28]

But here's where the story takes a particularly cynical turn: Rather than facing financial ruin for their role in creating this epidemic, pharmaceutical companies discovered they could profit from it twice—first by selling the drugs that cause addiction, then by selling the drugs to "treat" it.

This "double dip" represents one of the most egregious examples of profit-driven exploitation in medical history. Companies that made billions creating addiction now stand to make billions more from medication-assisted treatment, using drugs like buprenorphine, methadone and naltrexone to manage opioid dependence.

The pharmaceutical industry has played a massive role in both creating and sustaining the addiction crisis. First, they flooded the market with opioids, assuring doctors that drugs like OxyContin were "nonaddictive." When addiction rates skyrocketed, they turned around and sold the solution—expensive MATs (medication-assisted treatments).

Even Purdue Pharma, the company most directly responsible for igniting the opioid epidemic, attempted to cash in on the treatment side. In 2015, the company received a patent for a new version of buprenorphine and promptly sued another drug company, Indivior, for marketing a similar treatment.[29]

This isn't to suggest that MAT isn't valuable. When properly implemented, it can be lifesaving. The problem lies in how these medications are often deployed: as profit centers rather than components of comprehensive recovery programs.

MAT was designed to combine medications with counseling and behavioral therapies, hence the "assisted" in "medication-assisted treatment." Yet in practice, many programs simply distribute medications with minimal therapeutic support. Patients report meetings with doctors lasting mere minutes, with little to no counseling or addiction education provided.

The economic incentives behind this medication-only approach are clear: Dispensing pills is cheaper and more profitable than providing comprehensive therapy. A patient on maintenance medications represents a steady revenue stream that can continue for years or even decades without requiring the intensive staff resources that therapy demands.

This creates a troubling scenario where patients are kept in a state of managed dependency rather than supported toward full recovery. While some may need long-term medication support, many others are never given the opportunity to heal completely because doing so would terminate their value as ongoing customers.

The pharmaceutical industry has leveraged its political

influence to ensure this profitable arrangement continues. Between 2006 and 2015, pharmaceutical companies spent more than $880 million on lobbying and campaign contributions—nearly three times what the gun lobby spent during the same period.[30] This investment has paid off in favorable regulations, minimal oversight of marketing practices and continued protection from meaningful liability for their role in creating the opioid crisis.

Even as companies like Purdue Pharma, Johnson & Johnson, AmerisourceBergen, Cardinal Health and McKesson have agreed to pay billions in settlements, these amounts represent a fraction of the profits they reaped from selling addictive drugs. The $26 billion settlement reached in 2022 may sound substantial, but spread across multiple companies and years, it barely dents their bottom lines, and is even more insignificant when compared to the estimated $1.3 trillion economic impact of the opioid crisis over just two decades. [31]

Perhaps most disturbing is that these companies can effectively write off these settlements as business expenses, reducing their tax burden and further diminishing the financial consequences of their actions. Meanwhile, the human cost —hundreds of thousands of lives lost, millions of families devastated, entire communities hollowed out—can never be adequately compensated for.

The opioid crisis and its aftermath represent a case study in how profit motives can corrupt healthcare, transforming patients into commodities to be exploited rather than people to be healed. From creating addiction through deceptive marketing to profiting from partial treatments that maintain dependency, pharmaceutical companies have demonstrated a willingness to sacrifice public health on the altar of shareholder value.

When Numbers Lie: The Manipulation of Success Rates

"Our program has a success rate of 85%!"

"Nine out of 10 of our clients achieve lasting sobriety!"

"Our treatment approach is 75% effective!"

These bold claims plaster the websites, brochures and advertisements of addiction treatment centers across America. They offer hope to desperate families and individuals searching for solutions. There's just one problem: most are fundamentally misleading.

The manipulation of success rates in addiction treatment represents one of the industry's most ethically questionable practices. By exploiting inconsistent definitions, selective sampling and short follow-up periods, facilities create the illusion of effectiveness while obscuring the reality of their outcomes.

Let's decode how this statistical sleight of hand works.

First, there's the critical question of how "success" is defined. Many facilities count any client who completes their program as "successful," regardless of what happens afterward. It's akin to a university claiming a 100% success rate because no student skipped a class, regardless of whether they actually learned anything or graduated.

Others define success as abstinence at 30 days post-discharge, a woefully inadequate time frame for a chronic, relapsing condition. Given that the highest risk period for relapse is typically 30 to 90 days after treatment, these short-term measurements conveniently capture the brief "pink cloud" phase before the real challenges of recovery begin.

Then there's the matter of who gets counted. Many programs exclude clients who leave treatment early (against medical advice, or AMA) from their statistics, despite these individuals often representing 20 to 30% of admissions.[32] Others omit clients who relapse quickly after discharge, arguing they "weren't ready" for recovery and therefore shouldn't count against the program's effectiveness.

The result is a deeply skewed picture of treatment outcomes. As Dr. John F. Kelly, founder of the Recovery Research Institute at Harvard Medical School, explains: "Most treatment success rates are misleading because they don't follow patients long enough. Addiction is a chronic condition, and real success should be measured over years—not weeks."[33]

The manipulation extends to how data is collected. Many treatment centers rely on self-reporting through voluntary follow-up surveys, a method virtually guaranteed to produce inflated success rates, as those doing poorly are less likely to respond. Some facilities even count clients as "successful" if they simply cannot be reached for follow-up, assuming no news is good news.

As Dr. Kelly notes, "Most treatment success rates are misleading because they don't follow patients long enough," a reality confirmed by NIDA data showing that 40 to 60% of patients relapse within one year, with some studies suggesting 85 to 90% of traditional 30-day program completers return to substance use within 12 months.[34]

This discrepancy between marketing claims and reality doesn't just mislead consumers—it has profound consequences for treatment design and funding. When programs can hide their failures through statistical manipulation, they have little incentive to innovate or improve their approaches. Why invest in development if you can simply redefine success to make your current methods appear effective? Wouldn't it be a simple step in the right direction to regulate what kinds of statistics rehab centers are allowed to use in their marketing materials?

The deception also complicates insurance coverage. When insurers see inflated success rates for short-term programs, they have little motivation to cover longer, potentially more effective treatments. Why pay for 90 days if marketing materials suggest 30 days works 85% of the time?

But perhaps the most damaging impact is on patients themselves. When someone relapses after a treatment that claimed a 90% success rate, they don't question the program's effectiveness—they question their own worth. "Something's wrong with me" becomes the inevitable conclusion, deepening shame and making future recovery attempts even more challenging.

Some treatment centers defend their misleading statistics as "aspirational" or "motivational." They argue that giving clients hope, even false hope, serves a therapeutic purpose. But this rationalization ignores the ethical obligation of healthcare providers to obtain informed consent based on accurate information. Would we accept a cancer treatment that claimed a 90% cure rate when actual remission rates were 15%? Why do we accept such deception in addiction care?

The solution begins with standardized, transparent reporting of treatment outcomes. Programs should be required to track and disclose long-term results (minimum one to two years post-discharge), using consistent definitions of success, accounting for all admitted clients and employing rigorous follow-up methods that don't rely solely on voluntary responses.

Consumers deserve to know what they're buying. Families investing their life savings in treatment should understand the real probability of various outcomes. And people struggling with addiction need accurate information to make informed choices about their care.

Until the industry is held accountable for its claims, the gap between marketing promises and treatment reality will continue to trap vulnerable people in cycles of false hope, inevitable disappointment and deepening shame—all while treatment centers profit from the repeated "failures" they never honestly acknowledged were likely in the first place.

Breaking the Cycle: Toward an Ethical Treatment Model

Nathan's story is far from unique. Millions of Americans are caught in the revolving door of addiction treatment, bouncing between expensive programs that offer temporary respite but fail to provide the comprehensive care needed for lasting recovery. The system isn't merely failing; it's designed to fail in ways that generate continued revenue without delivering sustained healing.

Breaking this cycle requires a fundamental restructuring of the addiction treatment industry, one that aligns economic incentives with patient outcomes rather than patient returns. Here's what this transformation might look like:

1. **Payment models tied to outcomes, not services rendered.** Imagine a system where treatment centers receive full payment only when clients maintain recovery for one year or longer, with bonus payments for two and five years of continued success. This would rapidly shift focus from short-term stabilization to long-term healing.

Honestly, that doesn't seem like it would ever practically happen. But what if we try something a little easier?

2. **Improved outcome reporting.** Disallow rehab centers from using misleading statistics on their websites and marketing information. This forces them to prioritize referrals from clients, ensuring they commit to patient-centered approaches and focus on sustainable recovery.

3. **Regulatory requirements for transparent outcome reporting.** Treatment centers should be required to track and publish their actual

success rates using standardized measures across meaningful time frames (minimum one year post-discharge). Claims that cannot be substantiated with data should be prohibited as false advertising.

4. **Insurance coverage aligned with evidence.** The arbitrary 28-day coverage model should be replaced with flexible benefits that support the full continuum of care needed for brain healing: potentially 90 days or more of structured treatment, followed by step-down services that might extend 12 to 24 months.

5. **Diversification of treatment approaches.** The 12-step monopoly must give way to a customized treatment approach where treatment is matched to individual needs, so diverse patients are no longer forced into a one-size-fits-all model. This requires insurance coverage for proven alternatives like cognitive behavioral therapy, motivational enhancement therapy, contingency management and medication-assisted treatment with proven proper psychological support, along with many other evidence-based treatments.

6. **Accountability for pharmaceutical companies.** Manufacturers who profit from both creating and treating addiction should face meaningful financial penalties that exceed their profits from these practices. Settlement funds should be directed specifically toward developing effective, non-pharmaceutical approaches to addiction recovery and should include covered care costs for segments of the most affected populations, specifically impoverished and lower-income communities.

7. **Empowering consumers with the right questions.** For those researching treatment

centers for themselves or loved ones, asking the right questions can cut through marketing claims to reveal actual program quality.

Key Questions to Ask:

- What percentage of your patients complete your program, and what percentage of those completers are still sober 12 months post-discharge?
- How do you gather this follow-up information? Do you rely on voluntary surveys, or do you actively track outcomes?
- How long do your programs last, and what determines when someone is ready for discharge?
- Do you offer step-down programs or continuing outpatient services after initial treatment?

Red Flag Questions:

- Do you guarantee success? What is your success rate? If it's above 70 to 80%, that's a red flag.
- Are you licensed and accredited by recognized organizations? What are they and can I check? If not: another red flag.
- Do you allow prospective clients to speak with alumni or current participants? You already know what I'm going to say—if they say no, it's a red flag.

Such changes would not be popular with many stakeholders in the current system. Treatment centers would face greater accountability for their results. Insurance companies would initially face higher costs for comprehensive care (though they would likely see savings in the long run through reduced readmissions). Pharmaceutical companies would lose their lucrative "double dip" opportunity.

But these changes would transform the lives of millions caught in cycles of addiction and inadequate treatment. They would redirect billions of dollars currently wasted on ineffective interventions toward approaches that actually heal. And they would begin to address the massive public health crisis that addiction represents—a crisis that claims more American lives each year than were lost in the entire Vietnam War.

The current business model of addiction treatment isn't just ineffective; it's ethically indefensible. It exploits the vulnerable, profits from failure and perpetuates suffering that could be alleviated with existing knowledge and resources. We can and must do better.

In the next chapter, we'll explore how scientific neglect allows this profit-driven system to persist despite overwhelming evidence for better approaches.

3

Scientific Neglect: The Evidence Gap in Addiction Treatment

Your Brain on Recovery: What Science Actually Shows

Maya had been clean for exactly 27 days when the treatment center began preparing her discharge paperwork. She sat in the clinical director's office, feeling a fog of confusion that seemed to press against her skull like atmospheric pressure before a storm.

"How are you feeling about graduation, Maya?" the director asked, sliding the aftercare recommendations across the desk.

Maya searched for words. Simple decisions felt over-whelming: what to eat for breakfast, which route to take to group therapy. Even following conversations sometimes required extraordinary effort. But wasn't she supposed to feel better by now? Everyone kept talking about her "progress" and how "ready" she seemed.

"I'm grateful for everything," she said carefully. "But I'm wondering...is it normal to still feel so...cloudy? Like my brain isn't quite working right yet?"

The director nodded sympathetically. "That's very

34

common in early recovery. You'll find that attending meetings and working the steps will help clear that up. The important thing is that you've completed the program successfully."

Maya walked out with her completion certificate and a growing sense that something fundamental was being missed. Her brain felt like it was still rebooting from a massive system crash, yet somehow 28 days was supposed to be enough time for a complete restore.

What Maya didn't know—what no one had told her—was that cutting-edge neuroscience research shows her brain was exactly where it should be at 27 days: barely beginning the long journey of structural and functional recovery.

The disconnect between what neuroscience reveals about brain recovery and what treatment programs deliver represents one of the most profound failures in modern healthcare. While we can measure brain healing with unprecedented precision, most addiction treatment operates as if this science doesn't exist.

Dr. Judith Grisel, neuroscientist and author of *Never Enough: The Neuroscience and Experience of Addiction*, explains the biological reality of addiction: "The brain that got us into addiction is the same brain that has to get us out. But that brain needs time—real time, measured in months and years, not weeks—to rebuild the neural architecture that addiction dismantled."[35]

Neuroplasticity research demonstrates that the brain can reassign functions from damaged areas to healthy ones, but this reorganization requires sustained abstinence and appropriate environmental support. Recent neuroimaging studies reveal that significant brain changes can occur within weeks to months of abstinence, but complete rewiring can take a year or more.[36]

That timeline bears no resemblance to current treatment models:

- **Zero to 30 days:** Acute neurochemical stabilization begins. Executive function remains significantly impaired. Decision-making, impulse control and emotional regulation are at their most vulnerable. The brain experiences immediate changes, but withdrawal symptoms may manifest as the brain adjusts to the absence of addictive substances.
- **30 to 90 days:** Gray matter volume begins to recover in some regions, but neural connectivity remains fragmented. Individuals often experience improved mood and cognitive function, but the brain is still adjusting and the risk of relapse remains high. This is when most people are discharged from residential treatment.
- **90 to 180 days:** Dopamine receptor density shows measurable improvement. Working memory and attention begin meaningful recovery. The brain continues to heal, with many people noticing a reduction in cravings as neuroplasticity allows formation of new habits and behaviors.
- **Six to 24 months:** After six months to a year of abstinence, the brain has made significant progress in rewiring itself, though complete recovery can take longer, especially for those with severe or long-term addiction histories. This is when genuine neurological recovery reaches clinically significant levels.

The prefrontal cortex, the brain region responsible for executive function, decision-making and impulse control, shows the most dramatic deficits in early recovery and the slowest restoration. Research demonstrates that disruptions in three areas of the brain are particularly important in addiction: the basal ganglia, the extended amygdala and the prefrontal cortex. Yet treatment protocols routinely discharge patients when these critical systems are still profoundly impaired.

The evidence is overwhelming: Brains don't heal on insurance schedules. They heal on biological timelines that treatment centers either don't know about or choose to ignore. The question isn't whether we have the science to understand recovery—we do. The question is why we continue to build treatment systems that operate in complete opposition to what that science reveals.

The Fog Doesn't Lift in 30 Days: Understanding Post-Acute Withdrawal Syndrome

Marcus had been discharged from his third treatment program feeling optimistic. Twenty-eight days clean, completion certificate in hand, aftercare plan mapped out. But six weeks later, he sat in his sponsor's kitchen at 2 am, sobbing with frustration.

"I can't think straight," he whispered. "I forget things constantly. I start sentences and lose track of what I'm saying. Everyone keeps telling me I'm in a good place, but I feel like I'm losing my mind."

His sponsor, a man with 15 years of sobriety, nodded knowingly. "That's normal, brother. Just keep coming to meetings. The fog will lift."

But Marcus' fog wasn't lifting. If anything, it was getting thicker. What nobody, not his counselors, not his sponsor, not his aftercare therapist, understood was that Marcus was experiencing a well-documented neurological phenomenon that treatment programs systematically ignore: post-acute withdrawal syndrome.

PAWS represents one of the most critical gaps between addiction science and treatment practice. Post-acute withdrawal syndrome refers to a cluster of psychological and mood-related symptoms that can last for months to years after acute withdrawal from a substance, and it is a major contributing factor for relapse.

This isn't a theory or a hypothesis. Scientists believe that PAWS occurs as a result of the physical changes in the brain that take place during active substance abuse. The syndrome affects the majority of people in early recovery: 90% of recovering opioid users and 75% of recovering alcoholics will experience PAWS.[37]

Yet most treatment programs either don't acknowledge PAWS or dismiss it as part of "normal" early recovery without addressing its profound implications for relapse risk and treatment planning.

While acute withdrawal refers primarily to the body's process of healing, post-acute withdrawal syndrome occurs as the brain recalibrates after active addiction. The symptoms are neurological, not psychological:

- **Cognitive impairment:** Difficulty concentrating, memory problems, confusion and impaired decision-making. These aren't character flaws—they're measurable deficits in brain function.
- **Emotional dysregulation:** Anxiety, depression, mood swings and emotional numbness. The brain recalibration process takes anywhere from six months to two years before the brain once again naturally produces endorphins and dopamine.
- **Sleep disturbances:** Insomnia, vivid dreams and disrupted sleep cycles that can persist for months.
- **Physical symptoms:** Fatigue, coordination problems and sensitivity to stress that reflects ongoing neurological adaptation.

The timing of PAWS symptoms reveals the cruelty of 30-day treatment models. Post-acute withdrawal syndrome typically begins within seven to 14 days after completion of acute withdrawal, with symptoms that can persist for up to two years after stopping substance use. This means PAWS often peaks precisely when people are being discharged from treatment.

PAWS symptoms come and go and are usually triggered by stress, but are not constant misery. This intermittent nature makes the syndrome particularly insidious—people experience periods of clarity that make them believe they're "cured," followed by cognitive crashes that feel like regression.

Marcus' experience illustrates a tragic pattern: PAWS symptoms are routinely misinterpreted as psychological weakness, lack of motivation or resistance to recovery. In reality, they represent the brain's ongoing struggle to recalibrate systems that addiction fundamentally altered.

The research on PAWS reveals specific neurobiological mechanisms. The syndrome may be due to persisting physiological adaptations in the central nervous system manifested in the form of continuing but slowly reversible tolerance, disturbances in neurotransmitters and resultant hyperexcitability of neuronal pathways.

These aren't abstractions. They're measurable changes in brain chemistry and function that directly impact a person's ability to make decisions, regulate emotions and resist relapse. Yet treatment programs routinely discharge people at the height of these vulnerabilities.

Offering a prominent counter-perspective to the disease model is Dr. Lewis' *The Biology of Desire*. "We're asking people to make life-altering decisions and resist powerful cravings with brains that are still profoundly impaired. It's like asking someone to run a marathon with a broken leg and then blaming them when they collapse." [38]

The fog doesn't lift in 30 days because the brain doesn't

heal in 30 days. PAWS represents irrefutable evidence that addiction treatment timelines are based on economics, not neuroscience. Until we align treatment with brain healing rather than insurance billing, we'll continue to discharge people at their most vulnerable moment while calling it "graduation."

Evidence Ignored: The Research We're Not Using

The story of evidence-based addiction treatment is one of remarkable scientific progress systematically ignored by an industry invested in maintaining the status quo. We have decades of research demonstrating effective approaches that remain sidelined not because they don't work, but because they threaten the profitable simplicity of current models.

Dr. Kathleen Carroll's groundbreaking work at Yale University exemplifies this tragedy. Before her death in 2020, Dr. Carroll had spent nearly three decades developing and testing cognitive behavioral therapy approaches for addiction, establishing CBT as one of the most rigorously validated interventions in the field. Her research demonstrated that CBT produces significantly better outcomes than standard approaches, with effects that persist long after treatment ends. [39]

Carroll's team developed CBT4CBT—Computer Based Training for Cognitive Behavioral Therapy—which became one of the first evidence-based computerized interventions validated in multiple randomized clinical trials. The program teaches specific skills for identifying triggers, managing cravings and developing healthy coping mechanisms. In studies of cocaine-dependent patients, those who received CBT4CBT were more likely to achieve abstinence and used less cocaine during six-month follow-up periods.[40]

"CBT4CBT is now one of the only computer-based interventions demonstrated to be effective in multiple studies," Dr. Carroll noted. Her CBT manual for cocaine use disorders has been translated into over 14 languages and implemented worldwide, yet CBT remains relegated to "supplemental" status in most US treatment centers.

The evidence base extends far beyond CBT:

- **Contingency management** provides tangible rewards for verified abstinence and treatment engagement. Research consistently shows it's among the most effective interventions for stimulant use disorders, with some studies showing 40 to 60% abstinence rates.[41] Yet contingency management is rarely implemented because it requires infrastructure to provide rewards and verify abstinence through testing, complexity that many programs find inconvenient.

- **Medication-assisted treatment with comprehensive support** shows lifesaving efficacy when properly implemented. Research demonstrates that medications like buprenorphine and methadone significantly reduce mortality for opioid use disorders, but only when combined with comprehensive behavioral therapies.[42] However, providing comprehensive MAT requires medical staff, ongoing monitoring and integration of psychosocial services, investments many programs avoid.

- **Mindfulness-based relapse prevention** demonstrates effectiveness for preventing relapse, with brain imaging showing activation of regions that modulate emotion, self-regulation and interoception. Preliminary studies highlight its potential in addiction treatment, yet mindfulness-based interventions require specialized training and don't fit neatly into traditional group therapy formats.[43]

The pattern is clear: We have multiple evidence-based approaches that could dramatically improve outcomes, but they remain underutilized because they require investment in training, infrastructure and individualized care.

When researchers survey treatment centers nationwide, they consistently find that approximately 75% rely primarily on 12-step facilitation, with other approaches relegated to "supplemental" status or eliminated entirely due to cost considerations.[44] This isn't because 12-step approaches are more effective—the research shows they work about as well as other established treatments and help some people but not others.

The economic incentives work against the implementation of evidence-based approaches. A treatment center can run 12-step groups with minimal staff training and standardized materials. Implementing multiple evidence-based approaches requires investment in training, supervision and ongoing quality assurance.

Meanwhile, a major Cochrane review found that manual-ized 12-step facilitation programs can lead to *higher rates of continuous abstinence* compared to other treatments like CBT. However, for other metrics like reducing drinking intensity, they perform about the same. The key distinction is between peer-led AA and structured, therapist-led 12-Step Facilitation (TSF).[45]

Insurance companies compound the problem by reim-bursing programs for "treatment," rather than evidence-based treatment. A center receives the same payment whether they provide cutting-edge CBT or outdated confrontational approaches.

The result is a treatment landscape where evidence-based practices are often treated as expensive luxuries rather than standard care. People seeking help are told they're receiving "treatment" when they're actually receiving whatever approach the center finds most convenient and profitable to deliver.

Consider the research on personalized treatment matching. Studies consistently show that different approaches work better for different populations: CBT for those with trauma histories, motivational enhancement for those with ambivalence about change, contingency management for stimulant users, comprehensive medication-assisted treatment for opioid dependence.

But personalized matching requires assessment, flexibility and multiple treatment options. It's far simpler and cheaper to funnel everyone through the same program regardless of individual differences.

The most damaging aspect of this evidence gap isn't just that people don't receive optimal treatment; it's that they're told they've received "state-of-the-art" care when they've actually received approaches that research shows are less effective than available alternatives.

The tragedy isn't that we don't know what works—we do. The tragedy is that economic and institutional barriers prevent most people from accessing treatments that research shows are most likely to help them achieve lasting recovery.

When Old Science Trumps New: The Rejection of Emerging Research

While neuroscience advances at breakneck speed, addiction treatment practice remains anchored to models developed when our understanding of the brain was primitive. This resistance to emerging research represents one of the most troubling aspects of the addiction treatment field.

The resistance operates through several mechanisms that protect existing approaches from scientific scrutiny:

- **Appeal to tradition:** The argument that approaches are valid because they've been used for a long time, regardless of outcome data. The fact that 12-step programs were developed in 1935 becomes evidence for their effectiveness rather than a reason to question their relevance to modern neuroscience.
- **Anecdotal override:** Individual success stories are used to dismiss statistical evidence of poor outcomes. When presented with data showing 60 to 90% relapse rates, defenders point to the 10 to 40% who succeed as proof the approach works, ignoring the majority who don't benefit.
- **Moving goalposts:** When research challenges existing models, the definition of "success" shifts. If abstinence rates are poor, success becomes "engagement in the recovery process." If retention is low, success becomes "planting seeds for future recovery." With no standard definition of success, it becomes harder to determine what a particular treatment, rehab center or doctor is actually achieving.
- **Economic entrenchment:** Existing programs have invested heavily in infrastructure, training and marketing around particular approaches. Adopting new models would require admitting that current investments were suboptimal and committing resources to fundamental change.

Consider the emergence of neurofeedback and neuroplasticity-based interventions. Studies consistently show that people in early recovery have profound deficits in working memory, attention and executive function. Functional neuroimaging demonstrates specific deficits in prefrontal cortex function that correlate with relapse risk.

Cognitive training interventions directly address these deficits through targeted exercises that enhance neural connectivity and improve cognitive function. Brain imaging studies show measurable improvements in prefrontal cortex activity after training. Yet when treatment centers are presented with this research, the common response is: "That's interesting, but we focus on the spiritual aspect of recovery."

The irony is stunning. Centers reject scientifically validated brain training while embracing approaches with no neurobiological basis and poor outcome data.

The pattern repeats across emerging research areas:

- **Transcranial magnetic stimulation** (TMS) demonstrates potential for reducing cravings and enhancing executive function through targeted modulation of specific brain circuits. Evidence suggests TMS may be effective in diminishing substance use cravings by regulating activity in brain regions associated with addiction.[46] As a non-invasive neuromodulation procedure, TMS has shown efficacy in treating various mental health disorders, including depression, anxiety and post-traumatic stress disorder (PTSD). The TMS system market represents a growing sector within the mental health treatment landscape, though the technology continues to evolve as an emerging therapeutic modality.

- **Personalized medicine approaches** use genetic testing to identify individuals who metabolize medications differently or who have specific vulnerabilities that affect treatment response. This could revolutionize treatment matching, yet most centers continue one-size-fits-all approaches.

- **Virtual reality exposure therapy** allows
people to practice coping skills in simulated high-
risk environments, building resilience before facing
real-world triggers. Research shows promise for
superior outcomes compared to traditional
relapse prevention.[47]

Each of these approaches has solid research foundations
and addresses specific neurobiological aspects of addiction.
Yet they struggle for adoption while approaches with minimal
scientific support remain standard practice.

The institutional barriers are formidable. Treatment
centers operate under regulatory frameworks that emphasize
compliance with established standards rather than innovation.
Staff are trained in traditional approaches and resist methods
that challenge their expertise. Insurance reimbursement favors
familiar interventions over novel approaches.

Most importantly, the current system profits from failure.
If emerging interventions dramatically improved outcomes,
the revolving door business model would collapse. Centers
would lose repeat customers and face pressure to demonstrate
superior results.

Meanwhile, people seeking help receive 20th-century
interventions for a disorder that 21st-century neuroscience has
revolutionized our understanding of. The science exists. The
resistance is institutional, not empirical.

The Neuroscience Revolution at the Door: What Recovery Could Be

At research institutions across the country, a quiet revolution is taking place. Scientists are developing interventions that
directly target the neurobiological roots of addiction,
producing outcomes that traditional approaches can only
dream of achieving.

The transformation begins with precise diagnosis. Rather than relying on self-reported symptoms and behavioral observations, researchers are using detailed neuroimaging to map brain structure and function, revealing the extent of addiction-related damage and identifying which neural circuits need targeted intervention.

Major progress in genetics and neuroscience research has illuminated neurobiological processes that contribute to vulnerability for drug use and addiction, giving us understanding of the neurocircuitry disrupted in addiction. Treatment interventions intended to reverse these neuroadaptations show promise as therapeutic approaches for addiction.

Consider what's now possible with current neuroscience tools:

- **Assessment-driven treatment planning:** Instead of fitting people into predetermined programs, interventions are designed around neurobiological findings. Someone with severe executive function deficits receives intensive cognitive training. Someone with trauma-related amygdala hyperactivity gets targeted emotional regulation therapy. I've touched on this already and I'll delve deeper in later chapters: It's what we call "Customized Care."
- **Precision pharmacotherapy:** Genetic testing identifies how individuals metabolize medications, allowing personalized dosing and drug selection. Some people are rapid metabolizers who need higher doses; others are slow metabolizers at risk for toxicity. Traditional approaches use standard doses despite individual variations.
- **Targeted cognitive enhancement:** Brain training programs can improve specific deficits in working memory, attention and impulse control.

Molecular mechanisms underlying drug-induced brain plasticity can be targeted therapeutically, with neuroplasticity allowing formation of new neural connections crucial for recovery.

- **Biomarker-guided treatment:** Blood tests and brain imaging can predict relapse risk and guide intervention intensity. High-risk patients receive more intensive support; stable patients can safely step down to lower levels of care. Think about this for a moment: It's a time-saving, money-saving, treatment-enhancing step-down approach that includes not only a psychological assessment, but biological markers like blood evaluation and brain imaging. It's almost like we would be making decisions based on what we know instead of what we think—or worse yet, doing what we do because we have always done it that way.

- **Personalized trigger management:** Individual brain responses to specific cues can be mapped, allowing personalized relapse-prevention strategies. Someone whose brain shows strong reactivity to alcohol cues needs different preparation than someone who responds primarily to stress.

- **Real-time progress monitoring:** Brain imaging tracks actual neural changes rather than relying on subjective reports. Patients can see their brains healing, which provides powerful motivation and objective evidence of progress.

- **Flexible duration:** Treatment continues until neurobiological markers reach target levels rather than ending at arbitrary calendar dates. Some patients need 60 days; others need 200. The brain's healing timeline determines discharge, not insurance schedules. The adoption of this single

approach could change the face of
recovery permanently.

The economic case for neuroscience-based treatment is compelling. While initial costs are higher due to brain imaging and specialized interventions, long-term costs plummet because people actually recover rather than cycling through repeated treatments.

Let's imagine for a moment that brain imaging equipment is too expensive to be practical. What if we took a different approach—one that actively involves patients in their own recovery? Instead of passively sitting in therapy, patients could receive neuroscience-based training that teaches them how their brains actually work. I'm not talking about watching a YouTube video and discussing it in a group meeting. I mean bringing in someone with specialized expertise, someone who can guide patients in understanding the neural mechanisms behind addiction and recovery.

When patients grasp how their brain is wired and how it can rewire itself, they can take an active role in their own healing. They can practice strategies to influence their own brain chemistry, to retrain circuits and to reinforce healthy patterns. This approach shifts the model from "We, the experts, wave our magic wand while you sit there," to one where patients are empowered participants in the science of their own recovery.

Traditional treatment often feels like an endurance test; people struggle through days filled with group meetings, hoping willpower will overcome brain chemistry. Neuro-science-based treatment feels like healing; people watch their cognitive function improve, cravings diminish and emotional regulation strengthen. Think about how this will give them hope, embolden them and cause them to drive forward with faith they didn't previously have—faith in themselves, faith in something bigger than them and maybe even faith that someone or something is on their side.

This transformation isn't science fiction. It's happening now in research clinics and progressive treatment centers that have embraced neuroscience-guided practice. The technology exists. The research is robust. The outcomes are superior.

The barriers are institutional, not scientific. Treatment centers would need to invest in brain imaging equipment, train staff in neuroscience-based interventions and restructure programs around individual brain healing rather than standardized timelines.

Insurance companies would need to reimburse for longer, more intensive treatment that actually produces lasting results rather than cheaper interventions that require repeated use.

Most importantly, the field would need to acknowledge that addiction is fundamentally a brain disorder requiring brain-based solutions, not primarily a spiritual or behavioral problem requiring moral transformation.

The neuroscience revolution isn't coming—it's here. We just haven't allowed it through the doors of most treatment centers yet. But for those fortunate enough to access neuroscience-based care, the difference is transformative: Instead of managing a lifelong struggle, they're experiencing genuine brain healing and lasting recovery.

The question isn't whether neuroscience-based treatment works. The evidence for that is overwhelming. The question is how long we'll continue to withhold effective brain-based interventions while calling outdated approaches "treatment." For people struggling with addiction, the answer can mean the difference between a life of relapse and genuine healing.

Maya's fog began to clear not at 28 days, but at 127 days —exactly when neuroscience predicted it would. By then, she had long since graduated from a program that discharged her when her brain was still barely beginning its recovery journey. Marcus learned about PAWS through his own research, finally understanding that his cognitive struggles weren't personal failures but predictable neurobiological responses.

The late Dr. Carroll's CBT4CBT program continues to demonstrate favorable outcomes in research settings and has successfully transitioned from experimental investigation to clinical implementation. Licensed clinical professionals and approved healthcare agencies can purchase per-patient access for complete treatment courses. Neuroplasticity-based interventions show remarkable promise in specialized clinics while traditional centers continue operating as if the brain were a black box.

The science exists. The evidence is overwhelming. The only thing standing between current practice and truly effective treatment is our willingness to prioritize brain healing over institutional convenience, long-term recovery over short-term profits and scientific evidence over comfortable traditions.

The revolution in addiction treatment isn't coming. It's here.

4

Revolving Doors: Why Fragmented Care and Abstinence-Only Approaches Fail

The treatment system isn't designed to cure addiction; it's designed to keep people cycling through it. If rehab actually worked long-term, these centers would lose their most reliable source of income—repeat clients.

The Graduation Ceremony

William stared at the certificate in his hands, the gold letters spelling out "Certificate of Completion." Day 30. Around him, 12 other patients applauded as the program director smiled and shook each graduate's hand.

"Congratulations, William," Dr. Martinez said warmly. "You should be proud. You've worked hard these past four weeks."

William managed a smile, though something hollow echoed in his chest. The withdrawal symptoms were gone. His body had healed. The Suboxone had stabilized him. So why did he feel like he was standing at the edge of a cliff?

"I have some concerns," he said quietly. "I feel better physically, but the nightmares are still there. The panic attacks. I keep thinking about my ex-wife, about what she did to me. I don't feel like I have any tools for dealing with that stuff—the stuff that made me start using in the first place."

Dr. Martinez nodded sympathetically, glancing at his watch. "Recovery is a process, William. What you've accomplished here is huge—you've broken the physical dependence. That's the foundation everything else builds on. Your outpatient counselor will help you work through those other issues."

"But I don't have an outpatient counselor yet. The waiting list is six weeks long, and my insurance won't cover the trauma specialists."

"I'm sure something will work out," he said, his tone gentle but final. "You have the tools now. Trust the process."

Three hours later, William sat in his car, discharge paperwork spread across the passenger seat. The transition plan looked impressive: outpatient counseling (when available), NA meetings, follow-up with his primary care doctor (who knew nothing about addiction) and 30 days of Suboxone. What the paperwork didn't capture was the terror of returning to the apartment where he'd overdosed six weeks ago, to the isolation and trauma that had driven him to heroin in the first place.

The Biological Band-Aid: Why Detox Alone Fails

The first few weeks went better than expected. William attended meetings religiously, filled his time with recovery activities and stayed sober. But the nightmares were getting worse. Every night, he relived the three years of abuse that had driven him to seek oblivion in a needle. The program had taught him that addiction was a disease, that his only job was to not use drugs. But nobody had taught him how to live with the memories that felt like broken glass in his chest.

He was sober, but he wasn't recovering. He was just enduring.

Here's the uncomfortable truth about most addiction treatment: It's not actually treating addiction. It's treating withdrawal. The medical establishment has become so focused on managing the acute symptoms of substance dependence that they've forgotten addiction is fundamentally about what drives people to seek oblivion in the first place.

One study of detoxification programs found a 44% readmission rate for alcohol detox patients within one year. Another study found a 58.8% yearly readmission rate in a nationwide sample of alcohol detoxification patients.[48]

Think about that for a moment. We're discharging people from "treatment" when fewer than one in three will receive any continuing care. It's like performing emergency surgery, then sending the patient home without addressing the underlying condition that caused the issue.

William's experience illustrates the fundamental flaw in treating addiction as a primarily medical problem requiring medical solutions. Yes, detoxification is necessary. Yes, medication-assisted treatment can be lifesaving. But when medical stabilization becomes the end goal rather than the starting point, we've reduced human suffering to a chemistry problem.

Believe it or not, in some corners of the country, particularly where treatment resources are scarce or professionals are woefully undereducated, a dangerous delusion persists: that detoxification alone constitutes adequate addiction treatment. This magical thinking suggests that once the substances are flushed from someone's system, they'll somehow emerge transformed, equipped with the tools and insights necessary for sustained recovery. It's the medical equivalent of believing that cleaning a wound cures the underlying infection.

Yet this approach thrives, especially in regions where treatment centers are limited and among practitioners who mistake withdrawal management for comprehensive care. More cynically, some detox facilities have discovered that this "patch-and-release" model creates a lucrative revolving door where patients predictably relapse within weeks, generating repeat admissions and fresh insurance billing opportunities. The lesson couldn't be clearer—detox addresses sobriety, but sobriety is not recovery!

This means that brain chemistry matters. But the trauma that rewired that brain chemistry matters more.

The Graduation Illusion: The Danger of Day 30

When William finally got into outpatient treatment, Dr. Patel spent 30 minutes focused mainly on medication management. "How are you feeling on the Suboxone?" he asked, barely looking up from his computer.

"Fine, I guess, but I'm having trouble with anxiety and depression and—"

"That's normal in early recovery. We'll keep you on the current dose. Are you attending meetings?"

"Yes, but—"

"Good. I'll see you in two weeks."

Meanwhile, his primary care doctor knew nothing about addiction treatment. The trauma therapist he'd seen before treatment was no longer covered by insurance. The new specialists had waiting lists measured in months. William found himself caught between systems that didn't talk to each other, where each provider assumed someone else was handling what they weren't.

The "graduation ceremony" William experienced represents one of the most dangerous deceptions in addiction treatment: the illusion that completing a program equals readiness for independent recovery. Treatment centers have become remarkably skilled at reframing arbitrary insurance timelines as clinical milestones. (I've shared this in our clinics for years.) We, as professional treatment centers, fail our clients regularly by allowing them the false sense of security they have when leaving after an extended period of sobriety, more sobriety than they have experienced in, occasionally, 20 years or more.

This window of sobriety must be guarded sacredly by a case management team committed to constant follow-up and follow-through.

Day 30 has achieved almost mystical significance in addiction treatment despite having no basis in neuroscience, psychology or recovery research. The 30-day model emerged not from clinical evidence but from insurance reimbursement schedules designed in the 1970s and 1980s.[49] Yet somehow this billing convenience became enshrined as the gold standard for treatment duration.

The psychological impact of premature "graduation" is profound. Patients like William are told they're "ready" when their brains are still healing, their trauma remains unprocessed and their coping skills are largely theoretical. When they inevitably struggle, as neuroscience predicts they will, they're left believing the problem is their personal inadequacy rather than the treatment system's fundamental misunderstanding of recovery timelines.

White-Knuckling Through Sobriety: Why Abstinence Alone Isn't Recovery

By week six, William was drowning in bureaucracy and barely staying afloat emotionally. He was still sober, technically, but miserable, isolated and increasingly hopeless. The certificate on his wall felt like a cruel joke.

The relapse, when it came, felt almost inevitable. Fifty-three days, and William was back in the emergency room with a combination overdose that nearly killed him. The intake nurse looked at his chart with a mixture of pity and frustration. "Weren't you just in treatment?"

"I graduated," William whispered.

The addiction treatment field has developed an almost religious reverence for abstinence that borders on the absurd. Don't misunderstand—abstinence from addictive substances is typically necessary for recovery. But the field's obsession with counting days sober while ignoring quality of life has created a recovery culture that celebrates miserable sobriety as success.

Here's the problem with our obsession with counting sobriety days: It transforms recovery into a high-stakes game where a single misstep erases years of progress and personal growth. The neuroscience is clear on this point. This "all-or-nothing" mentality triggers what researchers call the abstinence violation effect, where the shame and perceived "failure" of a minor slip become the psychological fuel for a full-blown relapse.

Consider what happens when someone with three years of sobriety has "just one drink" and suddenly becomes a "new-comer" who has "lost all their time." We're not promoting accountability in these moments; we're weaponizing perfectionism against people whose brains are already wired for self-destruction.

Moreover, the ritual of day-counting creates a perverse dynamic. It keeps the DOC (drug of choice) at the center of someone's identity, keeping the substance at the forefront of their consciousness rather than allowing them to build a life where addiction becomes increasingly irrelevant.

Perhaps most damaging of all, the worse someone feels about themselves because of their using history, the less likely they are to refuse the next opportunity to use. This makes our shame-based counting system a self-fulfilling prophecy that keeps people trapped in cycles of relapse and self-recrimination.

William's experience highlights the critical distinction between sobriety and recovery. Sobriety is the absence of substance use. Recovery is the presence of a life worth living without substances. The current system excels at producing white-knuckle sobriety—tense, joyless abstinence maintained through willpower and fear—while failing spectacularly at fostering genuine recovery. Personally, I have encountered countless individuals who are technically sober but fundamentally miserable, people who traded one form of suffering for another while being told this constitutes success.

According to a 2020 study published in *The American Journal of Psychiatry*, the risk of fatal overdose is 10 to 40 times higher in the two weeks after discharge than at any other time. These aren't statistics about treatment failure; they're evidence of a system that discharges people at their moment of maximum vulnerability while calling it "graduation."[50]

Real recovery requires addressing the underlying drivers of addiction: trauma, mental health conditions, social isolation, lack of purpose and spiritual emptiness. When treatment focuses exclusively on removing substances without building a foundation for a meaningful life, it creates a recovery house built on sand.

The Handoff That Never Happens: The Gap Between Care Levels

As they wheeled William into the same detox unit he'd been in two months earlier, he realized he wasn't caught in a cycle of addiction—he was caught in a cycle of treatment that treated everything except the reasons he'd started using drugs in the first place. The system had taught him to be a patient, but it had never taught him to be a person, and certainly not a healthy person.

The mythology of "continuum of care" is one of the addiction treatment field's most persistent fantasies. On paper, the system appears comprehensive: Detox leads to residential treatment, which connects to intensive outpatient care, which transitions to ongoing support and monitoring. In reality, these levels of care operate as independent silos with minimal coordination and dangerous gaps between them.

William's experience navigating multiple uncoordinated providers represents the norm rather than the exception. His detox team didn't communicate with his residential program. His residential counselors had no contact with his outpatient providers. His outpatient psychiatrist knew nothing about his trauma history. His primary care doctor was flying blind about addiction treatment protocols.

This fragmentation isn't accidental. It's the predictable result of a system that prioritizes billing efficiency over treatment coordination. Each level of care operates as a separate profit center with its own documentation requirements, billing protocols and discharge criteria. Patient welfare becomes secondary to administrative convenience.

The human cost of this fragmentation is measured in lives lost during transitions. The highest-risk periods for overdose death occur not during active use, but during the gaps between treatment episodes when people fall through the cracks of uncoordinated care. We'll explore what true continuum of care looks like in Chapter 7.

Out the Door Too Soon: The Highest-Risk Moment

William's second hospitalization lasted three days, just long enough for medical stabilization before insurance coverage ended. This time, there was no graduation ceremony. No optimistic discharge planning. Just a social worker apologizing that the waiting list for residential treatment had grown to eight weeks.

"We'll get you on the list," she said, handing him a bus voucher and contact information for local meetings. "Try to stay safe until a bed opens up."

He walked out of the hospital at 11 am on a Tuesday, into a world where nothing had changed—except his tolerance had reset. The apartment where he'd overdosed. The dealers who knew his patterns. The trauma that had driven him to heroin in the first place. All waiting exactly where he'd left them.

The timing of treatment discharge reveals the profound disconnect between clinical need and operational convenience. Insurance authorizations end, beds become needed for new admissions and treatment programs measure success by completion rates rather than long-term outcomes.

According to data from the Substance Abuse and Mental Health Services Administration (SAMHSA), the average length of stay in residential treatment has dramatically decreased over the past three decades. This reduction occurred not because treatment became more effective, but because managed care organizations demanded shorter stays to control costs.[51]

As covered in the previous chapter, the neuroscience is unambiguous about recovery timelines. Healing the addicted brain requires months to years, not weeks. Executive function, impulse control and emotional regulation, the cognitive abilities essential for maintaining recovery, show measurable improvement only after 90 to 180 days of sustained abstinence. Yet we routinely discharge people when these critical systems are still profoundly impaired.

The phrase "out the door too soon" understates the magnitude of this problem. We're not just discharging people prematurely—we're actively sabotaging recovery by creating transitions that neuroscience tells us will likely fail.

Siloed Systems: When Right Hand Ignores Left

William's story doesn't end with relapse, though statistically, that's where most stories like his conclude. Fortunately, there are addiction specialists who operate differently. Instead of treating addiction as an isolated medical condition, these practitioners coordinate with trauma therapists, connect patients to peer support services and work with primary care doctors to create integrated treatment plans.

"Addiction isn't happening in a vacuum," explains one

such specialist. "We need to treat the whole person, not just the chemistry."

When patients receive this kind of coordinated care, they achieve something traditional programs rarely offer: recovery that feels sustainable because it addresses the wounds that drive addiction.

The tragedy of William's initial treatment experiences isn't that they were malicious—they were well-intentioned efforts operating within a fundamentally broken system. Each provider was competent within their narrow scope of practice. The failure occurred at the system level, where medical, psychological, social and spiritual aspects of recovery are treated in isolation rather than as integrated components of a complex condition.

True recovery requires what systems theorists call "horizontal integration," coordination across disciplines and providers to address addiction's multiple dimensions simultaneously. Instead, our current system offers "vertical fragmentation," where separate experts address separate aspects of the same problem without communication or coordination.

The irony is devastating: We've created specialists who are experts at treating parts of addiction while missing the addiction entirely. It's like assembling a team of specialists to treat heart disease—a cardiologist for the cardiovascular system, a nutritionist for diet and a kinesiologist for exercise—but never allowing them to speak to each other about the same patient.

William's recovery began only when someone finally saw his addiction as one manifestation of deeper wounds requiring coordinated healing and "Customized Care." Until the field embraces this integrated approach as standard practice rather than exceptional care, we'll continue recycling people through fragments of treatment while wondering why the whole remains broken.

The revolution in addiction treatment isn't coming from new medications or innovative therapies. It's coming from the radical idea that maybe, just maybe, we should treat people as whole human beings rather than collections of symptoms to be managed in isolation.

In the next chapter, we'll explore how the treatment system's failure to address trauma, family dynamics and cultural context creates additional barriers to lasting recovery, leaving entire dimensions of human experience unaddressed in the pursuit of healing.

5

The Whole Person Overlooked: Trauma, Family and Cultural Context

"The question is never 'Why the addiction?' but 'Why the pain?' Yet most treatment programs focus entirely on stopping the behavior while ignoring the emotional and spiritual emptiness that drives it."
—Dr. Gabor Maté

The Missing Piece: Trauma as the Template for Addiction

Marcus sat in the parking lot of the clinic, engine idling, staring at the small orange bottle in his palm. Day 127 on Suboxone. The physical cravings were manageable now. The medication had done its job there. But the nightmares were getting worse. Every night, he was back in that basement, age seven, listening to his stepfather's footsteps on the stairs.

In the clinic, Dr. Peterson would ask the same questions: "How are you feeling on the medication? Any cravings? Side effects?" The appointment would last 12 minutes, maybe 15 if Marcus mentioned sleep problems. Dr. Peterson would adjust the dosage, print a new prescription and send him on his way with a reminder to attend NA meetings.

What Dr. Peterson never asked about were the panic attacks that hit Marcus in crowded spaces. The way his heart raced when someone raised their voice. The hypervigilance that kept him scanning exits wherever he went. The crushing weight of shame that no amount of Suboxone could touch.

"The medication is working," Dr. Peterson had said last week, reviewing Marcus' clean drug screens. "Your recovery is on track."

But Marcus didn't feel like he was recovering. He felt like he was managing. The opioids had been his escape from memories that felt too big to carry. Now, sober and medicated, those memories sat in his chest like broken glass, sharp and unmoving. The Suboxone kept him from using, but it did nothing to heal the wounds that had driven him to heroin in the first place.

Marcus had tried bringing up the trauma before. "I think some of my using was connected to things that happened when I was a kid," he'd said during one appointment.

Dr. Peterson had nodded briefly. "That's what therapy is for. Focus on staying clean for now."

But the waiting list for trauma therapy was eight months long, and his insurance didn't cover specialists who understood both addiction and complex trauma. The system treated his addiction as if it existed in a vacuum—nothing but a brain disease requiring medication management—with no connection to the childhood terror that still lived in his nervous system.

As Marcus finally walked into the clinic for his appointment, he wondered how many others sat in this waiting room carrying wounds that medication alone could never heal. How many were told they were "recovering" while the deepest sources of their pain remained untouched?

The tragedy of Marcus' experience isn't unique. It represents the systematic failure of addiction treatment to address the underlying drivers of addictive behavior. Research reveals a staggering connection between trauma and substance use that most treatment programs systematically ignore. Studies show that up to 75% of people with substance use disorders have experienced significant trauma, yet the majority of treatment protocols focus exclusively on managing withdrawal and cravings while leaving emotional wounds to fester.[52]

As I wrote earlier, the landmark Adverse Childhood Experiences (ACE) study found that people with five or more adverse childhood experiences were 10 times more likely to develop substance addiction than those with none. Studies of treatment populations consistently find trauma rates of 60 to 90% among people seeking addiction treatment.[53] Yet somehow the addiction treatment field has constructed an elaborate system that treats the symptom while ignoring the disease.

Dr. Maté, one of the world's leading experts on addiction and trauma, explains the fundamental disconnect: "A hurt is at the center of all addictive behaviors. The wound may not be as deep and the ache not as excruciating, and it may even be entirely hidden, but it's there."[54] This isn't metaphorical language; it's neurobiological reality. Trauma creates measurable changes in brain structure and function that mirror many of the neurobiological alterations associated with addiction.

When children experience trauma, their developing brains adapt to survive in threatening environments. The stress response system becomes hyperactivated, the prefrontal cortex, which is responsible for executive function and emotional regulation, becomes impaired and the brain's reward pathways are altered. These same systems are disrupted by addictive substances, creating a neurobiologically perfect storm where substances become a logical solution to trauma-induced dysregulation.

For trauma survivors, substances aren't just recreational; they're medicinal. Genius Network founder and addiction recovery advocate Joe Polish reframes this relationship in a way that cuts through stigma and gets to the core truth: "I believe addiction is a solution [to a problem]."[55] This recognizes that people don't choose substances arbitrarily. They choose them because they work, at least temporarily, to solve the unbearable problem of emotional pain.

Polish explains that "the person struggling with addiction isn't weak or morally deficient," but a human being who found something that provided relief from suffering, even if that relief came with devastating consequences. Heroin doesn't just get you high; it stops the hypervigilance. Alcohol doesn't just provide relaxation; it silences the critical voice of an abusive parent that never stops echoing in your head. Cocaine doesn't just create euphoria; it temporarily fills the void left by childhood neglect. When someone discovers that a substance can provide relief from unbearable emotional pain, they've found what feels like a miracle cure. The problem isn't that it doesn't work, but that it works too well—until it doesn't work at all.

Yet most treatment programs operate as if this overwhelming evidence doesn't exist. They focus on removing substances without addressing why people needed them in the first place. It's like treating a person's lung cancer by confiscating their cigarettes while ignoring a tumor—technically accurate but fundamentally missing the point.

The consequences of this trauma-blind approach are measured in relapse rates that would be considered malpractice in any other medical field. When underlying emotional wounds remain unhealed, substances maintain their appeal as the most effective tool many people have found for managing psychological pain. No amount of medication or willpower can compete with the raw human need for relief from suffering.

Trauma-informed care represents a fundamental shift in how we understand addiction and approach treatment. Rather than asking "What's wrong with you?" trauma-informed approaches ask "What happened to you?" This simple reframing transforms addiction from a character defect requiring discipline into a survival strategy requiring healing.

True trauma-informed addiction treatment addresses both the neurobiological and psychological dimensions of recovery. It recognizes that healing involves not just managing cravings but developing new ways to regulate emotions, build safety in relationships and process experiences that were too over-whelming to integrate when they occurred. This work takes time—often months and even years, but certainly not weeks— and requires specialized training that most addiction coun-selors don't receive.

The evidence for trauma-informed approaches is compelling. Programs that integrate trauma treatment with addiction services show significantly better outcomes than traditional approaches, with higher retention rates, lower relapse rates and improved quality of life measures. Yet these programs are relegated to specialty clinics while the majority of people seeking help are shuffled through trauma-blind systems that address symptoms while ignoring causes.

Marcus' experience illustrates the human cost of this systematic neglect. His Suboxone prescription manages his opioid dependence effectively, he's no longer at risk of over-dose, no longer stealing to support his habit, no longer living the chaotic lifestyle that active addiction requires. By conven-tional measures, his treatment is successful.

But Marcus isn't living; he's enduring. The medication has removed one coping mechanism without replacing it with tools for managing the underlying distress that drove his substance use. He's trapped in a medical model that sees his brain chemistry as the problem and medication as the solu-tion, while the emotional wounds that created his vulnerability remain unacknowledged and untreated.

Until the addiction treatment field embraces trauma-informed care as standard practice rather than specialized intervention, we'll continue producing stories like

Marcus'—"successful" treatments that leave people sober but not healed, clean but not recovered, managing their addiction while the deeper sources of their suffering continue to drive them toward despair.

Medication Without Transformation: The False Promise of Quick Fixes

The billboard on Highway 101 promised hope in bold letters: "Get Your Life Back—Same Day Suboxone Appointments Available." Below the text, a smiling family embraced against a sunrise backdrop, suggesting the transformation that medication-assisted treatment could provide. For Marcus, driving past that billboard every day on his way to work, it represented both salvation and limitation.

What is MAT, you ask? Great question. Medication-assisted treatment uses three FDA-approved medications to treat opioid addiction: methadone, buprenorphine (Suboxone) and naltrexone (Vivitrol). These aren't substitutes for street drugs—they're precision tools that act on the same brain receptors targeted by opioids, but in fundamentally different ways.

Methadone and buprenorphine are opioid *agonists*: They bind to the brain's opioid receptors without producing euphoria, reducing cravings and preventing withdrawal while allowing normal brain function. Naltrexone, on the other hand, is an *antagonist*. It blocks those receptors entirely, making it impossible to get high from opioids.

Think of MAT as neurobiological armor: These medications either safely satisfy the brain's chemical needs (agonists) or protect it from opioid effects altogether (antagonists).

MAT has revolutionized addiction treatment in many ways. People with opioid use disorder (OUD) taking prescribed methadone or buprenorphine are less (59% and 38%, respectively) likely to die of overdose compared to those who receive no treatment. These medications stabilize brain chemistry, reduce cravings and provide a neurobiological foundation that makes recovery possible. When properly implemented, MAT is genuinely lifesaving.

But wait! Before you start thinking everything is rosy, there's a problem.

MAT programs don't always operate the way they're designed to.

The problem isn't with the medications themselves; it's how they're commonly deployed in a healthcare system that prizes efficiency over transformation. MAT provides a "whole-patient" approach to treat addiction to opioids such as heroin or prescription pain relievers. MAT is not a standalone treatment. It combines medications with behavioral therapy, different types of psychosocial support and other wraparound services. Yet in practice, many programs offer medication without the comprehensive support that makes MAT truly effective. To reiterate: the "M" in MAT is for "medication," the "A" is for "assisted" and the "T" is for "treatment." Notice that medication in this program is about assisting the treatment—it isn't meant to be the sole treatment itself.

So, if we're only using medication without therapy, we're not following the program as it was intended. In this scenario, we're essentially using drugs to avoid using drugs, a dangerous cycle I've seen play out countless times. A 2022 study in the *Journal of Substance Abuse Treatment* entitled "Psychosocial and behavioral therapy in conjunction with medication for opioid use disorder: Patterns, predictors, and association with buprenorphine treatment outcomes," found that 73.8% of buprenorphine patients received little to no therapy during services in the first six months of treatment, with an average of less than one day of therapy services per month.[56]

Dr. Daniel Amen, a psychiatrist who has scanned over 250,000 brains, advocates for comprehensive brain health approaches that address root causes rather than just symptoms.

While acknowledging that medications can help optimize brain function, he warns against treatments that focus solely on immediate symptom relief without addressing underlying issues, as this can lead to recurring problems. He emphasizes the importance of identifying and treating the root causes of mental health conditions through personalized, integrative approaches.[57]

The research supports the necessity of comprehensive care. A lack of availability of behavioral interventions is not sufficient justification to withhold medications to treat OUD, but studies consistently show that combining MAT with counseling and behavioral therapies produces superior outcomes to medication alone. Unfortunately, the reality of MAT delivery often falls far short of this ideal.

Marcus' experience reflects a pattern reported across the country: brief appointments focused primarily on medication management, minimal counseling support and little attention to the underlying factors that contributed to addiction. His 12-minute monthly appointments consisted mainly of reviewing side effects, checking for drug interactions and ensuring compliance with the medication regimen. When Marcus mentioned his trauma history, sleep problems or relationship difficulties, they were dismissed as issues for someone else to address.

This fragmented approach creates what some addiction specialists call "managed dependency," a state where people are stabilized on medications but never given the tools for comprehensive healing. While managed dependency is vastly preferable to active addiction, it represents a missed opportunity for genuine recovery rather than indefinite maintenance.

The economic incentives driving medication-only approaches are obvious. Dispensing pills requires less staff time, training and infrastructure than providing comprehensive therapy. A physician can see multiple MAT patients in the time it would take to conduct a single therapy session. From a business perspective, medication management is highly efficient and profitable. But efficiency isn't the same as effectiveness.

The human cost of medication-without-transformation approaches extends beyond individual outcomes. When people stabilize on MAT but don't receive comprehensive treatment, they often remain stuck in patterns of thinking, relating and coping that contributed to their addiction. Their relationships may improve somewhat due to the stability that medication provides, but underlying dynamics often remain unchanged. They may return to work or school, but without developing healthier stress management skills, they remain vulnerable to relapse if life becomes overwhelming.

More troubling is the fact that medication-only approaches can inadvertently reinforce the medical model's tendency to reduce complex human suffering to brain chemistry problems. When people are told that addiction is "just" a brain disease requiring medication, they may internalize the message that their emotional pain, relationship difficulties and spiritual emptiness are secondary concerns rather than core elements of their condition.

The alternative, comprehensive MAT that integrates medication with trauma-informed therapy, family work and psychosocial support requires a fundamental shift in how programs are structured and funded. It means longer appointments, ongoing therapeutic relationships and coordination between medical and behavioral health providers. It means acknowledging that healing from addiction involves more than stabilizing brain chemistry.

Neuroscience will agree that a mind that has been sober for a time makes better decisions. The key distinction is between MAT as a temporary stabilization measure and MAT as a permanent maintenance solution. When medications are used as a bridge to comprehensive treatment, providing the neurobiological stability needed for trauma therapy, family work and skill building, they can be transformative. When medications become the entirety of treatment, they may prevent overdose death while leaving people trapped in a form of recovery that feels more like management than healing.

Marcus' story continues to unfold. His Suboxone prescription has given him the stability to begin addressing the trauma that drove his heroin use, but only because he eventually found a program that understood medication as one component of comprehensive care rather than a complete solution. The transformation he experienced didn't come from the medication alone. It came from addressing the whole person rather than just brain chemistry.

For the thousands of people currently receiving medication-only MAT, the question isn't whether their treatment is valuable—it's whether it could be *transformative* with the addition of trauma-informed therapy, family support and psychosocial interventions. The medications are working exactly as designed. The tragedy is that we're settling for stabilization when healing is possible.

The Family Factor: When Treatment Ignores the System

When Marcus was finally admitted to a residential treatment program that understood trauma, the intake coordinator asked him an unexpected question: "Who else in your family has been affected by your addiction?"

Marcus paused, surprised. In three previous treatment episodes, no one had ever asked about his family beyond basic emergency contact information. His mother, who had watched him struggle with addiction for eight years, had never been invited to participate in his treatment. His teenage sister, who had learned to lock her bedroom door when Marcus was using, had never been offered support or education about addiction. His stepfather, the source of much of Marcus' trauma, was a painful absence that treatment programs had never acknowledged.

"My whole family," Marcus finally answered. "But nobody's ever asked about them before."

The systematic exclusion of families from addiction treatment represents another one of the field's significant oversights. When mothers seek substance use treatment, programming generally excludes their children, even though including children in the treatment process has the potential to positively impact their mothers' substance use outcomes, as well as improve parent-child interaction. Research consistently demonstrates that family members benefit just from learning about addiction, recovery and ways to respond to a family member's substance misuse, yet most programs treat addiction as if it occurs in a relational vacuum.[58]

This exclusion stems partly from confidentiality concerns and partly from the medical model's focus on individual pathology. Treatment centers worry about privacy violations and complex family dynamics that might complicate individual therapy. While the industry is right to have that concern, it's a challenge we can tackle with some intentionality and purpose. However, it's simpler to treat the "identified patient" without dealing with the messy realities of family systems where addiction typically develops and where recovery must ultimately be sustained.

But addiction doesn't respect family boundaries. Addiction is a family disease, according to the National Council on Alcoholism and Drug Dependence. It affects every member of the family and can cause deep dysfunction in the family system. [59] When one person develops an addiction, the entire family system reorganizes around the crisis, often in ways that inadvertently maintain the problem they're trying to solve. Without proper attention, this leads to multigenerational addictions.

Family members of people with addiction develop their own survival strategies: hypervigilance, emotional withdrawal, caretaking behaviors or even their own substance use. Children in addicted families learn to be silent about family secrets, to manage adult emotions and to expect disappointment. Spouses learn to control what they can and to manage crises that feel unpredictable. These adaptations make sense within the context of living with addiction, but they can become barriers to recovery if they're not addressed.

The research on family systems and addiction recovery is unambiguous. Family systems therapy has shown itself to be a powerful adjunct to substance use treatment for couples and for adolescent substance users. Studies consistently find that including family members in treatment improves retention rates, reduces relapse risk and enhances long-term outcomes for both the person with addiction and other family members. [60]

When people change their behavior in treatment but return to family systems that haven't changed, the mismatch can actually undermine recovery. Old patterns of interaction can trigger familiar emotional states that previously led to substance use.

Marcus' family had spent eight years organizing their lives around his addiction. His mother had learned to sleep with her car keys hidden so Marcus couldn't steal her car during binges. His sister had developed anxiety that kept her awake at night while she listened for sounds that might indicate Marcus was using. Family gatherings had become minefields of unspoken tension, with relatives walking on eggshells to avoid triggering conflict.

Many families often include enablers: people who, despite their best intentions, actually help maintain the addiction by removing consequences or making it easier for the addicted person to continue using. In Marcus' case, his mother had become the classic enabler. She paid his rent when he spent his money on drugs, made excuses to his employer when he missed work and even drove him to "doctor's appointments" that were actually visits to his dealer. She told herself she was helping him, protecting him from hitting rock bottom. But what she was really doing was preventing him from experiencing the natural consequences of his choices. The enabler often suffers from their own form of addiction, an addiction to being needed, to fixing, to controlling the uncontrollable. And they hide this addiction behind the mother of all emotions—love. *I do it because I love them.*

When Marcus completed his 30-day program, he returned to a family system that hadn't received any support, education or therapeutic intervention. His family wanted to be supportive but didn't know how. They were afraid to set boundaries that might trigger relapse, but also resentful about past hurt that had never been addressed. They loved Marcus but didn't trust him, creating a relational environment that was emotionally unsafe for everyone involved.

Family therapy aims to create a stable and calm home environment that will support the recovery of the addicted family member. This work involves more than educating family members about addiction—it requires addressing the relational patterns that developed during active addiction and building new ways of communicating, setting boundaries and providing support.

Effective family work in addiction treatment serves multiple functions. It helps family members understand addiction as a complex condition rather than a choice, reducing blame and shame that can interfere with recovery. It teaches communication skills that allow for honest conversation about difficult topics. It addresses enabling behaviors that may inadvertently support continued substance use. Most importantly, it helps the family system reorganize around recovery rather than addiction.

The evidence supports specific approaches to family involvement. Goals include engaging family members in treatment, providing information, enhancing social support networks, developing problem-solving and communication skills and providing ongoing support and referrals to other community-based services. This isn't about family therapy as it's traditionally understood, but systemic interventions that address addiction as a family-level problem requiring family-level solutions. This type of supportive family counseling tends to "normalize" the addiction or the addicted person. When family members come to understand the nature of their loved one's addictive challenges, they develop compassion, have less resentment toward them and better understand that addictive time in their loved one's life. This begins a healing process which, in my experience, is almost always necessary for recovery.

For Marcus, the breakthrough came when his treatment program offered family week, an intensive intervention that brought his mother and sister into the therapeutic process. For the first time, they were given vocabulary for describing their experiences. They learned about trauma's impact on brain development and how it contributed to Marcus' addiction. They practiced new ways of communicating that didn't involve either enabling or punishment.

Most importantly, they began to address the elephant in the room: the family's relationship with Marcus' stepfather, whose abuse had created the trauma that led to addiction. This wasn't about blame or reopening old wounds; it was about acknowledging realities that had shaped the family system and making conscious choices about how to move forward.

The transformation wasn't immediate or complete. Families don't reorganize overnight, and trust isn't rebuilt with good intentions alone. But for the first time in years, Marcus felt like he was returning to a family that understood addiction and had tools for supporting recovery rather than inadvertently undermining it.

The tragedy is that most families never receive this

support. They're left to navigate recovery with the same dysfunctional patterns that developed during active addiction, often leading to relapse cycles that could be prevented with appropriate family intervention. Many researchers have stressed the importance of involving family members in the treatment of substance users, as it can have a positive impact on relapse, retention and overall treatment outcomes.

The barriers to family involvement aren't insurmountable. They require treatment programs that expand the family's understanding of who the "patient" is, the development of staff competencies in family systems work and the structuring of programming that accommodates family participation. They require insurance systems that recognize family therapy as essential rather than optional. Most importantly, they require abandoning the myth that addiction is an individual problem requiring individual solutions rather than a customized problem requiring customized solutions.

Marcus' recovery gained momentum not just because he addressed his trauma, but because his family learned to support healing rather than pathology. When treatment programs exclude families, they miss the opportunity to transform entire systems rather than just individuals. In a field struggling with high relapse rates, this represents a systematic failure to address one of the most powerful factors influencing long-term recovery success.

Cultural Blindness: When Context Gets Erased

Maria Spotted Horse sat in the intake office of the urban treatment center, filling out forms that had no boxes for her reality. Race/ethnicity options included "Native American/Alaska Native," but nothing captured the complexity of being a Lakota woman navigating addiction treatment in a system built around concepts that felt foreign to her worldview.

The treatment counselor, a well-meaning white woman named Jennifer, reviewed Maria's paperwork with professional efficiency. "I see you marked that you're interested in spiritual counseling," Jennifer said. "We have an excellent chaplain here who leads our meditation groups."

Maria hesitated. How could she explain that her relationship with spirituality had been shaped by boarding school trauma, by ancestors who were punished for practicing traditional ceremonies and by a complex relationship with both Christian and Indigenous beliefs that no chaplain trained in Western traditions could understand?

"The meditation is based on mindfulness practices," Jennifer continued, "and we integrate the 12-step program throughout treatment. You'll find the spiritual principles very helpful."

Maria nodded politely, but inside she felt the familiar disconnection that came from being squeezed into frameworks that hadn't been designed for her experience. The 12-step program's emphasis on powerlessness contradicted everything her grandmother had taught her about reclaiming strength from historical trauma, and the individual focus of Western therapy ignored the collective healing that her culture understood as essential for true recovery.

Maria's experience reflects a pervasive problem in addiction treatment: the systematic erasure of cultural context. Most treatment programs operate from an unexamined assumption that addiction and recovery are universal experiences that can be addressed through standardized interventions. This cultural blindness creates barriers to treatment engagement and undermines the effectiveness of interventions that ignore the cultural factors that shape both addiction development and recovery pathways.

The statistics reveal the scope of this problem. Indigenous peoples experience addiction rates significantly higher than the general population, yet treatment completion rates are lower.[61][62] African American and Latino populations face substantial barriers to accessing treatment, and when they do engage, they often encounter programs that don't reflect their cultural values or address their specific experiences of discrimination and historical trauma.

Cultural factors influence every aspect of addiction and recovery. They shape how symptoms are understood and expressed, how families respond to addiction, what kinds of help-seeking are acceptable and what recovery means within their cultural context. They determine whether spiritual practices are seen as resources or problems, whether collective or individual healing is prioritized and whether traditional healers are viewed as allies or obstacles to treatment.[63]

For Indigenous communities, addiction often represents a symptom of historical or multigenerational trauma, which is informed by the cumulative emotional and psychological wounds transmitted across generations through systemic oppression, forced assimilation and cultural destruction. Boarding schools, Indian removal policies and decades of cultural suppression created what researchers call "soul wounds" that continue to impact Indigenous families and communities today.

Traditional healing approaches in Indigenous cultures emphasize the restoration of balance, maintaining a connection to community and land and addressing the spiritual as well as physical dimensions of illness. Recovery isn't seen as an individual achievement but as a return to cultural identity and community connection. These approaches have shown remarkable effectiveness when properly implemented and supported.[64]

Yet most mainstream treatment programs know nothing about multigenerational trauma, traditional healing practices or the cultural factors that influence addiction in Indigenous communities. They offer generic spiritual counseling instead of culturally specific healing practices. They emphasize individual accountability rather than community restoration. They pathologize cultural practices as "enabling" when they might actually be resources for recovery.

The situation is similarly complex for other communities of color. African American families dealing with addiction must navigate not only the stigma of substance use but also the additional burden of racial discrimination within health-care systems. The crack cocaine epidemic of the 1980s led to criminalization patterns that still affect how Black families view addiction treatment. Many approach treatment centers with justified suspicion about whether they'll receive compassionate care or judgmental intervention.[65]

Latino families often face language barriers, immigration concerns and incompatibilities with cultural values around family privacy that can interfere with traditional treatment approaches. Religious beliefs, family hierarchies and gender roles all influence how Latino families understand addiction and what kinds of interventions feel acceptable.[66]

LGBTQ+ individuals face their own cultural challenges in addiction treatment. Many treatment programs operate from heteronormative assumptions that ignore the specific stressors faced by sexual and gender minorities. The concept of "family" may not include chosen family members who provide crucial support. Religious-based treatment programs may be actively hostile to LGBTQ+ identities, creating additional trauma rather than healing.[67]

The research on culturally responsive treatment is clear: Programs that adapt their approaches to reflect cultural values and address culture-specific factors achieve better outcomes than generic programs. Culturally adapted interventions show higher retention rates, better treatment engagement and improved long-term outcomes across multiple populations.

But cultural responsiveness requires more than superficial accommodations. It's not enough to hang diverse artwork on the walls or hire bilingual staff if the underlying treatment philosophy remains unchanged. True cultural responsiveness requires understanding how culture shapes every aspect of addiction and recovery, from symptom presentation to help-seeking patterns to definitions of healing.

For Maria Spotted Horse, recovery began when she found a treatment program that understood multigenerational trauma and incorporated traditional healing practices alongside evidence-based treatment. The program was led by Indigenous clinicians who understood the connection between cultural disconnection and addiction, who saw traditional ceremonies as therapeutic interventions rather than obstacles to treatment.

The healing lodge where Maria eventually found recovery looked nothing like the sterile medical facility where she'd first sought help. It incorporated sweat lodge ceremonies, talking circles, connection to traditional foods, land-based activities and elder involvement in the healing process. The focus wasn't on individual pathology but on cultural reclamation and community restoration.

This approach didn't reject evidence-based treatment—it integrated cognitive behavioral therapy, trauma treatment and other proven interventions within a cultural framework that made them meaningful and accessible. The result was treatment that addressed not just Maria's addiction but the cultural and historical factors that had contributed to her vulnerability.

The implications extend beyond individual treatment outcomes. When treatment programs ignore cultural factors, they perpetuate health disparities that affect entire communities. They fail to address the social determinants of addiction that disproportionately impact communities of color. They miss opportunities to engage traditional healing resources that could strengthen treatment effectiveness.

Cultural blindness in addiction treatment isn't just insensitive; it's clinically incompetent. It represents a failure to understand that effective treatment must address the whole person within their cultural context. Until the addiction treatment field develops genuine cultural responsiveness, it will continue to fail the very communities that most need effective intervention.

Maria's story has a different ending than Marcus' not because her addiction was less severe or her trauma less significant, but because she eventually found treatment that honored her cultural identity rather than requiring her to abandon it. Her recovery involved reclaiming traditional practices that had been suppressed by multigenerational trauma, reconnecting with cultural identity that had been fragmented by assimilation and finding healing approaches, in the classroom and in the wilderness, that addressed both individual and collective wounds.

The revolution in addiction treatment won't just be about incorporating new technologies or evidence-based practices; it will be about creating space for multiple ways of knowing, healing and being that reflect the cultural diversity of people seeking recovery. Until treatment programs learn to see culture as a resource rather than a barrier, they'll continue to reproduce the very systems of oppression that contribute to addiction in the first place.

The stories of Marcus and Maria illustrate a fundamental truth about addiction treatment: Healing requires addressing the whole person within their relational and cultural context. When treatment focuses only on brain chemistry while ignoring trauma, family dynamics and cultural factors, it may achieve technical sobriety while missing the deeper transformation that makes recovery sustainable.

The neuroscience of addiction is real and important. Medications like Suboxone and methadone save lives and provide crucial neurobiological stability. Evidence-based therapies work. But they work best when implemented within comprehensive approaches that honor the complexity of human experience rather than reducing it to symptoms and diagnoses.

The future of addiction treatment lies not in choosing between medical and psychosocial approaches, but in integrating them within frameworks that address biological, psychological, social and cultural dimensions of recovery. This requires treating trauma as a core component rather than a secondary concern, engaging families as partners rather than obstacles and embracing cultural diversity as a source of healing wisdom rather than a complication to be managed.

Until we learn to see addiction within its full human context—as a response to wounds that require healing rather than symptoms that require management—we'll continue to produce stories like Marcus' early treatment experiences: "successful" interventions that leave people sober but not whole, clean but not healed, managing their addiction while the deeper sources of their suffering remain unaddressed.

The revolution in addiction treatment isn't coming from new medications or innovative technologies, but from the radical recognition that addiction happens to whole people embedded in families, communities and cultures that must all be part of the healing process. The question isn't whether we have the tools for this kind of comprehensive treatment. We do. The question is whether we have the wisdom to use them.

In the next chapter, we'll explore how systemic barriers determine who gets access to these tools and who remains trapped in inadequate interventions, and reveal how addiction treatment has become a tale of two systems where privilege determines the quality of care received.

6

Access and Equity: Who Gets Help and Who Doesn't

The uncomfortable truth is that your ZIP code, your skin color and your bank account balance are often better predictors of the quality of addiction treatment you'll receive than the severity of your condition.

The Tale of Two Recoveries

Samantha stared at her phone screen, scrolling through treatment center websites at 2 am. Her 17-year-old son Miguel had been using fentanyl for eight months, and tonight's overdose, his second in three weeks, had finally broken through her denial. The paramedics had saved him, but barely.

As a single mother working two jobs with basic Medicaid coverage, Samantha's options were limited. The first treatment center was encouraging until they ran her coverage. "We don't accept Medicaid for our residential program," the intake coordinator explained. "But we can put Miguel on our outpatient waiting list. The next opening is in six weeks."

Six weeks. Miguel might not survive six days.

By dawn, Samantha had called 14 facilities. The message

was consistent: Quality treatment required private insurance or cash payment she didn't have.

Meanwhile, across the city, Jennifer was having a very different experience. Her 18-year-old daughter Brittany had been struggling with cocaine and prescription pills, but Jennifer's husband carried premium insurance through his law firm.

"We can admit Brittany today," the admissions coordinator told Jennifer during their consultation in the center's mahogany-paneled office. "Our 90-day program includes individual therapy, family counseling, equine therapy and wilderness therapy. Your out-of-pocket cost will be about $25,000 for the full program."

Jennifer winced but nodded. They'd refinance the house if necessary.

Both Miguel and Brittany were 18 years old with supportive families desperate to help them recover. But their ZIP codes, insurance coverage and family income determined whether they received world-class treatment or were warehoused until the next crisis.

This isn't a story about personal responsibility. It's about how systemic barriers create a two-tiered treatment system where privilege determines not just access to care, but the quality of care received.

The Two-Tiered System: Quality Care for the Privileged Few

The addiction treatment landscape in America resembles a luxury cruise ship where first-class passengers dine on gourmet meals while steerage passengers fight for scraps. The difference isn't just in amenities; it's in outcomes, safety and the fundamental quality of care provided.

At the high end, private treatment centers market themselves as healing sanctuaries. Rolling hills, private chefs, massage therapy and individual counseling sessions with master's-level therapists. These facilities often maintain staff-to-patient ratios of two or three to one, allowing for intensive, personalized attention.

Brittany experienced this level of care. Her daily schedule included individual therapy, group counseling, family sessions, recreational therapy and wellness activities. When she struggled with anxiety in her third week, the center brought in a trauma specialist and extended her stay at no additional cost. Their philosophy was simple: Treatment continues until healing occurs, not until payment stops.

The contrast with publicly funded facilities couldn't be starker. These centers operate under severe financial constraints, often maintaining staff-to-patient ratios of one to five or lower. Counselors frequently hold only bachelor's degrees, and turnover rates often exceed 40% annually.[68]

Miguel eventually found placement at a converted motel 40 minutes from his home where 12 patients shared two bathrooms. His "counselor" was a well-meaning man with six months of sobriety and a weekend certification course. Group therapy sessions included 25 patients at once.

When Miguel experienced panic attacks, a common withdrawal symptom, the facility's response was to increase his anxiety medication and warn him that another "incident" would result in discharge. There was no trauma specialist, no individual therapy and no flexibility in his treatment plan.

Studies consistently show that facilities with higher staff-to-patient ratios, longer treatment durations and evidence-based programming achieve significantly better results.[69]

But perhaps most troubling is how the two-tiered system affects patients' sense of worth. Brittany left treatment feeling valued and equipped with tools for recovery. Miguel left feeling like a burden and a failure. When he relapsed six weeks after discharge, he internalized shame rather than recognizing he'd received inadequate care.

The tragedy isn't that luxury treatment centers exist, it's that basic quality care isn't available to everyone who needs it. We've normalized a system where your insurance card determines whether you receive evidence-based treatment or are simply processed through minimal care.

Insurance Barriers: When Coverage Decides Your Recovery

While Samantha struggled to find treatment for Miguel, James faced different but equally challenging barriers in rural Montana. A member of the Blackfeet Nation, James had insurance through the Indian Health Service, which technically covered addiction treatment. But the nearest IHS-contracted facility was 200 miles away, required a six-month wait and offered generic programming with no cultural relevance.

"They treat addiction like it's the same for everyone," James explained to his sister. "They don't understand that for us, this isn't just about stopping drugs. It's about healing from generations of trauma and reconnecting with our culture."

Insurance barriers manifest differently across populations, creating a complex web of access disparities that compound existing inequalities.

For elderly Americans, Medicare coverage remains limited. Dorothy, a 68-year-old retired teacher, developed an addiction to prescription opioids after surgery. Medicare would cover brief detox but not the extended therapy needed to address her depression and chronic pain.

"They want to treat her like she's a college kid who partied too hard," her daughter complained. "She needs specialized care for older adults, but Medicare won't pay for anything that sophisticated."

LGBTQ+ individuals face insurance barriers compounded by discrimination. Thomas, a transgender man, found that while his insurance covered addiction treatment, no covered facilities offered specialized programming for transgender patients. The closest LGBTQ+-affirming program was 500 miles away and not covered.

"I had to choose between living in housing that matched my gender identity or accessing treatment at all," Thomas said. He went without treatment for eight additional months while navigating insurance approvals, a delay that resulted in two more overdoses.

Rural populations face perhaps the most severe barriers. Sarah, a farmer's wife in Nebraska, had insurance that technically covered treatment. But the nearest facility was 180 miles away, and her policy didn't include provisions for housing or childcare during treatment.

"They told me I could get help, but I'd have to leave my farm and children," Sarah said. "That's not really coverage, that's abandonment."

Even ostensibly good insurance creates impossible choices. Many plans limit treatment to 30 days regardless of medical necessity, require extensive pre-authorization or exclude specialized care entirely. The prior authorization process alone creates significant barriers, as patients in crisis can't wait weeks for approval.[70]

Insurance companies frequently classify evidence-based treatments as "experimental," denying coverage for interventions proven effective. Trauma therapy, family counseling and extended care programs are often excluded despite research showing they improve outcomes.[71]

The result is a system where insurance coverage functions as a sorting mechanism that channels different populations toward different qualities of treatment. Those with premium coverage access comprehensive care. Those with basic coverage receive generic interventions. Those without coverage receive emergency interventions at best.

James eventually found recovery through a traditional

healing program run by tribal elders, funded through grants and tribal resources. "Real healing happened when I could be treated as a whole person, not just a diagnosis," he reflected. "But I shouldn't have had to choose between culturally appropriate care and insurance coverage."

The Language of Stigma: Labels That Keep People Suffering

Miguel was sitting in the emergency room when he overheard the attending physician talking to a nurse: "We've got another frequent flyer in bed seven. Typical junkie, probably here for drug-seeking behavior again."

Miguel felt his face burn with shame. He wasn't seeking drugs; he was seeking help. But the language used to describe him reduced his complex struggle to a dismissive label that painted him as manipulative rather than suffering.

The power of language in healthcare cannot be overstated, but the problem extends far beyond medical settings. Media, movies and social platforms have created a global narrative that portrays addiction as a unique moral failing affecting only certain "types" of people. This narrative ignores a fundamental truth: Addiction is the human condition.

The Universal Addiction We Refuse to Acknowledge

Dr. Joe Dispenza's groundbreaking research reveals an uncomfortable reality: We are all addicted. "People become addicted to the stress hormones, to those emotions. And then they need the bad job, they need the bad relationship, they need the traffic, they need the news just so that they can stay in that same emotional state," Dr. Dispenza explains. When we constantly live "under the gun of the fight or flight response, we mobilize an enormous amount of the body's energy for some threat in our lives, real or imagined."[72]

This stress hormone addiction affects millions who would never identify as having an addiction problem. Think of the executive who can't function without crisis, the parent addicted to perfectionism or the teenager dependent on social media validation. Research shows that an estimated 210 million people worldwide suffer from addiction to social media and the internet, while countless others compulsively chase stress chemicals through overwork, drama or perpetual busyness.[73]

Yet society reserves its stigma for substances while ignoring behavioral addictions that dominate modern life. We applaud workaholism while demonizing drug use. We normalize social media obsession while criminalizing chemical dependency. This selective moral judgment creates a hierarchy of addiction that serves no one.

Media's Manufactured Mythology

Movies and television have weaponized this selective stigma, creating powerful mythologies about who "addicts" are. Research consistently shows that media portrayals significantly influence public perception, often depicting people with substance use disorders through harmful stereotypes: the "tragic hero," "demonized user" or "comedic relief."[74] These simplistic characterizations bear little resemblance to reality but powerfully shape how society views addiction.

When celebrities reveal addiction struggles, coverage often focuses on their dramatic collapse rather than the complex factors underlying their dependency. Meanwhile, the same media celebrates figures who exhibit clear addictive behaviors around work, perfectionism or social media—without applying similar labels.

A study analyzing addiction portrayal in popular media found that 98% of movies contain depictions of substance use, yet most either glamorize consumption or demonize users.[75] Rarely do they explore addiction as a logical response to trauma, pain or the addictive nature of modern life itself.

Breaking the Hierarchy of Shame

Here's a revealing observation about human nature: You can put someone struggling with alcoholism in a room with a person addicted to methamphetamine, a person addicted to pornography, a person addicted to gambling and a person addicted to fentanyl, and they'll all look at each other as equals. They recognize their shared struggle.

But place a workaholic in that same room, or someone clearly addicted to stress, whose outlet is gaming, and they'll look down their noses at the others as if they aren't just as broken. This hierarchy of acceptable versus unacceptable addictions creates the very stigma that prevents healing.

Dr. John F. Kelly's research demonstrates that healthcare providers are significantly more likely to recommend punitive rather than therapeutic interventions when patients are described as "substance abusers" versus "people with substance use disorder."[76] But the language problem extends beyond clinical settings into everyday conversations where addiction terminology carries moral judgment.

Consider how different substances and behaviors are discussed. Prescription opioid dependency among middle-class populations is often described as an "epidemic" requiring "treatment" and "compassion." Social media addiction gets reframed as a "digital wellness challenge." Work addiction becomes "high achievement." Yet illegal drug dependency is labeled as "crime" requiring "punishment."

The same neurochemical processes drive all addictive behaviors. Whether someone compulsively checks Instagram, stays late at work to chase deadline adrenaline or uses heroin to escape trauma, the brain's reward circuitry operates identically. The only difference is societal approval of the substance or behavior.

The Path Forward: Universal Recognition

The solution isn't to shame everyone equally; it's to recognize addiction as a universal human experience that takes different forms. When we acknowledge that everyone has something they use to regulate emotions, manage stress or escape pain, addiction becomes a shared human condition rather than a character defect. I said it before: Addiction is customized to the individual. Therefore, recovery must be customized to the individual too.

Miguel eventually found recovery in a program that used person-first language and treated addiction as a health condition. "The first time someone called me 'a person with substance use disorder' instead of 'an addict,' I felt like they saw me as human," he reflected. "But what really changed everything was realizing that my counselor struggled with work addiction, my doctor was dependent on perfectionism and my sponsor had been addicted to controlling others. We were all just people trying to feel better."

True stigma reduction happens when society stops pretending that substance addiction is fundamentally different from the stress, perfectionism, social media, work and drama addictions that dominate modern life. We all have our substances. Some are just more socially acceptable than others.

Recovery advocacy organizations have promoted person-first language that emphasizes humanity before condition. But perhaps the most powerful destigmatization comes from recognizing that the person struggling with addiction isn't fundamentally different from anyone else; they're just using a different substance to manage the universal human experience of emotional pain.

"Did you create another problem by becoming addicted?"

"Yes, but that wasn't the intent; the intent was to manage the pain. Addiction was simply the consequence of my pain management choice."

When we stop dividing the world into "addicts" and "normal people," we create space for the truth: We're all trying to regulate our internal chemistry, and some methods just happen to be legal and socially acceptable, while some are not. This recognition doesn't excuse harmful behavior, but it creates the compassion necessary for effective treatment and genuine recovery.

From Patient to Criminal: The Justice System's Revolving Door

Three weeks after his last overdose, Miguel found himself in a police station rather than a treatment center. He'd been caught with a small amount of fentanyl for personal use, but any amount was classified as a felony. The arresting officer chose enforcement over emergency medical care.

"You're looking at two to five years," the public defender explained. "Or you can take a plea deal for 18 months if you agree to enter intensive probation."

Samantha stared in disbelief. Her son needed medical treatment for a chronic condition, but the system was offering prison and probation that treated addiction as a criminal justice problem rather than a health issue.

The criminalization of addiction represents one of the most significant barriers to treatment access. Rather than directing people toward healthcare, the justice system creates a parallel track that prevents access to evidence-based treatment while imposing additional barriers through criminal records, employment restrictions and social stigma.

In Miguel's story, probation illustrates how criminal justice approaches fail to address addiction as a medical condition.

While participants avoid prison, they're subjected to a punitive model emphasizing surveillance and punishment for relapse rather than individualized medical treatment.

Miguel's probation required twice-weekly court appearances, random drug testing, community service and group meetings that resembled probation check-ins more than therapy. Any positive drug test resulted in immediate jail time.

"They told me recovery was about personal responsibility and following rules," Miguel explained. "But nobody addressed why I was using drugs. They treated symptoms of my addiction like crimes instead of treating addiction like a disease."

This fundamentally misunderstands addiction science. Research demonstrates that stress is the biggest driver of addictive relapse and behavior.[77] Yet probation treats relapse as a violation worthy of punishment rather than a medical event requiring treatment adjustment, making recovery less likely, not more.

Criminalization affects different populations unequally. Communities of color are disproportionately arrested and prosecuted for drug-related offenses, despite similar substance use rates across racial groups.

James experienced this when arrested during active addiction. As a Native American man, he was more likely to be prosecuted harshly and less likely to be offered diversion programs compared to white defendants.

"They saw me as a criminal first, an Indian second and a person with a disease maybe never," James reflected.

Criminal records create long-term barriers extending beyond legal consequences. Employment discrimination limits economic opportunities supporting stable recovery. Housing restrictions prevent access to safe living situations. Educational barriers block pathways to advancement.

These collateral consequences often prove more destructive than the addiction itself. Miguel's felony record prevented him from accessing financial aid for community college, eliminated him from most entry-level jobs and created housing barriers, all factors that increase relapse risk. The cruel irony: People released from incarceration face a 40-times higher risk of overdose death than the general population, largely due to these systemic barriers.[78]

Dr. Maté explains the destructive cycle: "The addict is retraumatized over and over again by ostracism, harassment, dire poverty, disease, the frantic hunt for a source of the substance of dependence, the violence of the underground drug world and harsh chastisement at the hands of the law, all consequences of the war on drugs."[79]

International comparisons demonstrate that criminalization is a policy choice. Portugal's decriminalization model redirects people with drug-related offenses to health services rather than criminal courts, resulting in dramatic reductions in overdose deaths, HIV infections and drug-related crime.[80]

Some US jurisdictions have implemented reforms prioritizing treatment over incarceration. Seattle's Law Enforcement Assisted Diversion program allows police to refer people directly to treatment services rather than jail. Participants show significant reductions in recidivism and substantial increases in health service engagement.[81]

However, these programs remain exceptions. Most jurisdictions continue criminalizing addiction while expressing concern about overdose deaths, a contradiction reflecting the fundamental failure to align policy with scientific understanding.

Miguel eventually accessed effective treatment after completing drug court requirements and dealing with ongoing criminal record consequences. He now advocates for others caught in the justice system's web.

"Nobody should have to choose between medical treatment and avoiding prison," Miguel argues. "Addiction is a disease, not a crime."

A Path to Recovery: The Promise of Drug Courts

While the traditional criminal justice system often criminalizes addiction, leading to cycles of incarceration, a more progressive alternative has emerged: drug courts. These specialized courts represent a crucial diversion program, aiming to steer individuals with substance use disorders away from punitive measures and toward supervised treatment and rehabilitation. The first drug court was established in Miami, Florida in 1989, and since then, they have grown into a widespread movement across the United States, serving tens of thousands annually.[82]

When implemented with fidelity to their core principles, drug courts offer a powerful counter-narrative to the "lock 'em up" mentality. They provide immediate access to comprehensive treatment, including individual and group therapy, and often connect participants with vital supportive services like education, housing and employment assistance. This holistic approach recognizes that addiction is a complex health issue, not merely a moral failing, and that sustainable recovery requires addressing the underlying factors contributing to substance use. The intensive supervision, frequent drug testing and consistent judicial oversight inherent in these programs foster accountability while simultaneously providing a robust support system. This model has proven remarkably effective in reducing recidivism; studies consistently show that participants are significantly less likely to be rearrested compared to those processed through traditional courts.

Beyond the profound impact on individual lives, drug courts also deliver substantial societal benefits. They represent a fiscally responsible progressive alternative to imprisonment, yielding significant cost savings by reducing incarceration expenses and other criminal justice burdens. Studies show that for every dollar invested, the return on investment can range from over $2 to as much as $27 in societal benefits.[83] This economic efficiency, coupled with their capacity to transform individuals into productive, contributing members of society, underscores their value as both a public health and public safety intervention.

However, it's important to acknowledge that the effectiveness of drug courts is not uniform. Their success hinges on adherence to best practices, including robust clinical services, strong judicial leadership and a collaborative team approach. When these elements are compromised, drug courts can fall short of their potential, sometimes mirroring the punitive aspects of the traditional system or failing to provide truly evidence-based care. Yet when operated as intended, with a steadfast commitment to treatment, rehabilitation and the understanding that recovery is a process, not a single event, drug courts stand as a testament to the idea that compassion and accountability can converge to create profoundly favorable results for individuals, families and communities.

The Wild West of Rehab: When Anyone Can Open a Treatment Center

Six months into recovery, Miguel received a glossy brochure advertising a "revolutionary treatment center" in Florida. The marketing promised "luxury accommodations," "90% success rates" and "breakthrough therapies not available anywhere else."

What the brochure didn't mention was that the facility's "medical director" was a former plastic surgeon with no addiction training, that their "breakthrough therapy" consisted of unproven experimental procedures and that their "90% success rate" counted anyone completing their program as "successful," regardless of whether they remained sober afterward.

Unlike other healthcare areas with strict licensing requirements and quality standards, the addiction treatment industry operates with minimal regulation. In many states, virtually anyone can open a treatment center with little more than a business license. Medical supervision may be minimal. Staff qualifications often go unchecked. Treatment approaches can range from evidence-based medicine to pure quackery.[84]

This regulatory vacuum has created what industry insiders call the "Wild West of Rehab," a landscape where legitimate providers operate alongside unscrupulous operators who view addiction as a profit opportunity rather than a medical condition.

The consequences fall most heavily on vulnerable populations. People in crisis can't research options thoroughly. Families desperate to save loved ones may not recognize warning signs of predatory facilities. People with limited resources may be particularly susceptible to programs promising unrealistic outcomes at attractive prices.

Some operators exploit insurance regulations by providing minimal services while billing for comprehensive care. "Patient brokering" schemes pay recruiters to identify people with good insurance coverage and direct them to facilities that maximize billing rather than patient outcomes.

The Florida treatment industry became notorious for "body brokering" scandals where operators recruited people with addiction from across the country with promises of free treatment, then cycled them through multiple facilities to maximize insurance billing while providing minimal care.[85]

A significant scandal erupted in Arizona's addiction recovery sector, centered on the AHCCCS program, with major revelations emerging in May 2023. This elaborate fraud involved providers illicitly billing the state for an estimated $2.8 billion in unprovided or substandard addiction treatment, often preying on Native American individuals.[86] The crisis exposed how individuals were lured into fraudulent sober living homes, sometimes with tragic consequences, underscoring the devastating impact of unchecked exploitation within the behavioral health industry.

James encountered exploitation when seeking culturally appropriate treatment. A facility marketed itself as specializing in "Native American healing traditions." When he arrived, their "cultural programming" consisted of burning sage purchased online and "talking circles" led by staff with no tribal affiliation.

"They were selling my culture back to me as a marketing gimmick," James explained. "They took sacred traditions and turned them into props for their business model."

Thomas discovered similar deception at a program advertising "inclusive care for all identities." Despite inclusive marketing materials, staff had received no LGBTQ+ training, and Thomas faced daily microaggressions from both staff and other patients.

The lack of regulation enables false advertising about treatment approaches and success rates. Facilities routinely claim 80 to 90% success rates without defining "success" or providing supporting data. They may advertise "evidence-based treatment" for approaches that contain no scientific validation.

Quality treatment providers support stronger oversight, recognizing that substandard facilities damage the field's reputation while harming vulnerable patients. However, implementing meaningful regulation requires political will that often conflicts with industry lobbying and ideological opposition to government oversight.

Warning signs of problematic facilities include guarantees of success, refusal to accept insurance, pressure to sign contracts immediately, lack of medical supervision, unlicensed staff and promises of "miracle cures."

Miguel ultimately found effective treatment through a facility accredited by the Joint Commission and licensed by his state's health department. The center provided transparent information about their approach, staff qualifications and actual outcome data.

"The difference was night and day," Miguel reflected. "The legitimate facility treated me like a patient deserving quality care. The other places treated me like a customer they could take advantage of."

Breaking Down the Barriers: A Call for Equity

As Miguel approaches his second year of recovery, he's become an advocate for others facing the same barriers that nearly cost him his life. Working with a peer support organization, he helps families navigate insurance requirements, treatment options and systemic obstacles.

"Every week, I meet someone whose story sounds just like mine," Miguel explains. "Different details, same system failures. People dying not because treatment doesn't work, but because they can't access it."

The barriers documented in this chapter, such as economic disparities, insurance limitations, stigmatizing language, criminalization and regulatory failures, don't exist in isolation. They interact and compound, creating nearly insurmountable obstacles for those who most need help.

The opening observation bears repeating: "Your ZIP code, your skin color and your bank account balance are often better predictors of the quality of addiction treatment you'll receive than the severity of your condition." This represents a fundamental failure of a healthcare system that claims to treat addiction as a medical condition while maintaining barriers unthinkable for other diseases.

True equity means that Miguel and Brittany would receive the same quality of care regardless of insurance coverage or family income. It means that James could access culturally appropriate treatment that honors his Indigenous identity. It means that Marcus could receive affirming care addressing both his addiction and the minority stress that contributed to it.

Most importantly, equity means that Samantha wouldn't have to spend sleepless nights calling dozens of treatment centers, hoping to find someone willing to help her son before his next overdose becomes his last.

The barriers to addiction treatment represent moral failures as much as policy failures. They reflect a society that has decided, through action and inaction, that some lives are worth saving while others are acceptable losses.

Miguel survived these barriers, but barely. His recovery represents both individual resilience and the random luck of eventually connecting with competent, caring providers. Thousands of others don't survive long enough to find such care.

The revolution in addiction treatment won't be complete until every person struggling with substance use can access the same quality of care currently available only to the privileged few. This isn't just a healthcare imperative; it's a moral obligation to recognize the fundamental dignity of every human being seeking healing.

7

Treatment Reimagined: A New Paradigm for Addiction Recovery

The addiction treatment industry stands at a crossroads. After decades of documented failure, with relapse rates that would embarrass any other medical specialty, we finally have a choice: continue propping up a system that manages symptoms while people die, or build something that actually works.

This isn't another incremental improvement proposal. We're not talking about adding yoga classes or switching to organic meals, though both might help. We're talking about fundamentally reimagining how treatment organizations operate, from their foundational assumptions about human potential to the metrics they use to define success.

The transformation required isn't theoretical. The research exists, the methods are proven and the technology is available. What's been missing is a comprehensive blueprint that treatment providers can actually implement without going bankrupt or losing their licenses. This chapter provides that blueprint, along with some uncomfortable truths about why change has been so slow.

A handful of pioneering facilities have begun implementing elements of this new paradigm, proving that extraordinary outcomes are possible when we stop making excuses and start making changes. But these remain the rare exceptions. The goal is to make them the standard, not the anomalies that get featured in industry newsletters and then quickly forgotten.

The solutions presented here build directly on everything we've established in previous chapters. In Chapter 1, we demonstrated why different approaches work for different populations and established that treatment must be matched to individual needs rather than forcing people into predetermined models, recognizing that different individuals require different approaches based on trauma history, brain chemistry, psychological makeup, social context and personal values. Chapter 2 exposed the financial exploitation inherent in arbitrary 28-day coverage models and outlined the need for transparent outcome reporting, flexible benefits supporting the full continuum of care and potentially 90+ days of structured treatment followed by 12 to 24 months of step-down services. Chapter 3 revealed how treatment should align with brain healing timelines of six to 24 months rather than insurance schedules, continuing until neurobiological markers reach targets rather than arbitrary dates, while providing comprehensive medication-assisted treatment with behavioral therapies. Chapter 4 emphasized treating the whole person rather than just their chemistry, addressing addiction's multiple dimensions simultaneously through a true continuum of care with actual coordination between levels. Chapter 5 highlighted addressing trauma as a core component through trauma-informed care, comprehensive family work and culturally adapted interventions that reflect cultural values and address multigenerational trauma. Finally, in Chapter 6, we established that every person struggling with substance use should have access to the same quality care regardless of insurance coverage or family income, while implementing person-first language that treats addiction as a health condition rather than a moral failing.

This chapter will weave these elements together into a coherent system that serves the people it claims to help and maybe, just maybe, keeps them alive long enough to recover.

Section 1: The Foundation—Safety and Connection

Before any meaningful healing can occur, two fundamental conditions must exist: safety and connection. Without safety, people remain hypervigilant, unable to access the vulnerability required for therapeutic work. Without connection, both to the natural world and to other human beings, the isolation that drives addictive behavior persists even within treatment settings. Remember that addiction lives in secret, in the closet, in isolation, in places where nobody knows and nobody goes. The opposite conditions must be met in order for things to change.

The truth is most treatment environments, despite good intentions and expensive mission statements, inadvertently recreate the exact conditions that foster addiction, disconnection, powerlessness and emotional insecurity. Then we act surprised when people relapse.

Hari's insight that "the opposite of addiction isn't sobriety —it's connection" points to something crucial that most treatment centers miss entirely: You cannot treat addiction in isolation. Yet walk into most facilities and you'll find people isolated in individual rooms, isolated from their families, isolated from nature and often isolated from any sense of hope that things might actually get better.

The Two Faces of Safety

Safety operates on two critical levels that most centers completely ignore: patient-to-staff relations and patient-to-patient interactions. When either breaks down, the consequences are identical. People stop opening up, stop being honest in individual sessions and retreat into the protective patterns that addiction originally provided. In other words, they start planning their relapse.

Patient-to-staff safety centers on a deceptively simple question: Are team members treating patients as full human beings worthy of respect, or as problems to be managed until their insurance runs out? Are they demonstrating genuine compassion and understanding for the constant struggle that recovery represents, or are they going through the motions of "therapeutic communication" they learned in graduate school?

Tone of voice, body language and seemingly innocent questions can either invite vulnerability or trigger defensive responses faster than you can say "treatment plan." Most staff have no idea of the effect these things can have on patients because nobody taught them how hypervigilant nervous systems actually work.

Here's something that should be obvious but apparently isn't: Many individuals entering treatment are actually re-entering treatment. They arrive with preconceptions about how they'll be treated based on previous experiences not just in treatment facilities, but in interactions with law enforcement, court systems, frustrated family members and judgmental healthcare providers who act like addiction is contagious.

This presents an incredible opportunity that most centers completely waste. Instead of assuming people don't know what to expect, create the kind of loving, open environment that contradicts every assumption they have about how people in recovery are typically treated. This is one of the easiest and least expensive ways to improve outcomes, yet most centers are too busy arguing with insurance companies to notice.

Creating Environments That Actually Heal

Physical environment design plays a healthy role in establishing safety, though you'd never know it from visiting most treatment centers, which tend to look like they were designed by someone who confused "sterile" with "healing." Natural lighting, comfortable seating arrangements that allow for easy exit (because trapped animals don't heal) and spaces that feel more like homes than institutions all contribute to nervous system regulation.

Some facilities have discovered that incorporating plants, water features and natural materials can significantly reduce stress responses and promote healing. Others have discovered that fluorescent lighting and institutional furniture can trigger trauma responses. Guess which approach costs more and which one actually works?

The most critical element, however, is staffing. Treatment centers should prioritize hiring professionals who have personal experience with recovery, understanding that lived experience provides insights and credibility that cannot be gained through education alone. This isn't about discrimination against people without addiction histories; it's about recognizing that credibility in addiction treatment often comes from having walked the walk, not just memorizing the textbook and getting an A on the exam.

These staff members serve as living proof that recovery is possible while bringing an understanding of the recovery process that can only come from having experienced the hellish journey personally. When someone in early recovery sees staff members who have successfully navigated the same path, it provides hope and practical wisdom that can't be taught in any graduate program. And don't kid yourself about this one: How many of your patients sit across the desk from you or in the classroom and ask the question "What the hell does this person know about my addiction?" or "Why should I listen to them?" Relatability goes a long way in this conversation about safety and connection—don't you dare think it doesn't.

Staff training must extend far beyond traditional clinical skills to include trauma-informed communication, de-escalation techniques and cultural competency. Every team member, from clinical staff to kitchen personnel, should understand how to recognize signs of trauma activation and respond in ways that promote safety rather than retraumatization. This includes understanding how seemingly innocent questions like "What brings you here?" can trigger shame spirals in someone who's been asked that question by judges, probation officers and disapproving relatives for years.

The Power of Peer Connection

Patient-to-patient safety revolves around building genuine camaraderie and mutual support throughout the treatment community. The question isn't whether residents are following rules; it's whether they're helping each other, respecting each other's space and working together toward common goals. This isn't achieved through behavior contracts and point systems but by designing programs where patient-to-patient interaction becomes essential to daily functioning. It's worth saying again: This should be a primary focus for all client-facing staff on a daily basis.

Examples of fostering these kinds of interactions include structured activities that require collaboration, group projects that build on previous weeks' classroom teachings and service opportunities where residents work together to create authentic opportunities for healthy relationship building. When individuals work together to solve problems, overcome challenges or serve others, they develop genuine bonds based on shared experience and mutual support rather than shared misery.

The three foundational elements that distinguish truly transformative treatment environments are discipline, mutual respect and personal ownership. These concepts work synergistically to create communities where healing can flourish while maintaining the structure necessary for recovery. Get this wrong and you've created either chaos or a prison. Get it right and you've created something magical.

Discipline in this context differs fundamentally from the punitive control measures that most treatment centers mistake for structure. Instead of external rules enforced through threats and consequences, this methodology represents the cultivation of self-discipline and internal motivation that individuals need to sustain recovery beyond treatment.

This includes consistent routines that help people rebuild their relationship with time, responsibility and commitment, with consistent wake-up times, structured meals, therapy sessions and activities that help individuals experience the satisfaction that comes from following through on commitments to themselves and their community. It's about learning that structure creates freedom, not restriction.

When implemented well, this kind of discipline fosters personal ownership and mutual respect. People begin holding themselves, and each other, to higher standards. The shift is subtle but profound: Discipline moves from something enforced externally to something internally motivated. That's when real transformation begins. Individuals begin making healthy choices because they want to, not because they are being compelled.

And this matters deeply—not for you as a service provider, but for them. Your job is to step back and let them take responsibility for their own growth. This is where health takes root: when a person begins to believe, perhaps for the first time, that they can do this for themselves.

Mutual respect is the foundation of every healthy treatment community. It means that every person, regardless of their history, the severity of their addiction or their current struggles, is treated with dignity and worth. Respect is not something they earn by complying or improving. It is given because it is a basic human right. Staff model this through everyday interactions: disagreeing without degrading, setting boundaries without punishment and maintaining profession-alism while demonstrating real care.

It helps to look at a practical example of where many programs miss an opportunity: the kitchen. In a lot of centers, meals are prepared entirely by staff. The reasoning is sound; nutrition in recovery matters, and trained chefs and dietitians can ensure it. But when patients don't participate, a critical growth opportunity disappears.

Instead, imagine a dietitian overseeing a kitchen staffed by patients. They cook for each other, troubleshoot, organize and support one another. That's where teamwork and camaraderie emerge. Now picture a group of newer patients doing the dishes, cleaning the floors—knowing the person who prepared the meal started right where they are. They can see progress in front of them. They can feel possibility. The environment becomes not just therapeutic, but deeply safe and humanizing.

And, as a bonus, you no longer need a full kitchen staff.

Communication Standards That Actually Matter

Communication protocols within safety-focused treatment centers should emphasize transparency, respect and collabora-tion. Staff members need training to explain procedures before implementing them, ask permission before entering personal space and respond to resistance with curiosity rather than confrontation. These seemingly small changes in communication style can have profound impacts on an indi-vidual's sense of safety and willingness to engage authentically.

Respectful communication might mean establishing clear

standards around language use. Do you have consequences in place for the use of profanity or disrespectful language? You should. We all know which words we're referring to, and pretending that language doesn't matter is naive at best and harmful at worst. These standards aren't about controlling people; they're about creating environments where everyone feels safe to be vulnerable and where behaviors begin to change.

The creation of peer support networks within treatment settings provides another crucial element of safety. When individuals see others who share similar experiences and struggles, they begin to understand that they're not alone in their pain or their journey toward healing. Peer support groups, mentorship programs and informal community-building activities all contribute to the sense of belonging and acceptance that is essential for feeling safe enough to be vulnerable.

Alumni programs can work in connection with these peer support networks, creating ongoing opportunities for connection and growth that extend far beyond formal treatment completion. These programs create virtuous cycles where those who have found recovery become resources and inspiration for those still seeking it.

Nature and Connection: The Missing Piece

Integrating nature-based interventions addresses fundamental human needs often overlooked in traditional clinical settings. The therapeutic effects of natural environments are well-documented: Time in nature reduces cortisol levels, lowers blood pressure, improves immune function and supports mood regulation. For people in recovery, these benefits matter deeply because they speak directly to the stress responses and emotional dysregulation that fuel addictive behavior. For treatment centers working to create safer, more supportive environments, a meaningful connection to nature can be transformative.

However, wilderness activities should never be done "just to get outside." If you are going to invest the time and resources to take people outdoors, the experience must be purposeful. Think of outdoor programming as an extension of clinical work, not a break from it. Design activities that reinforce therapeutic lessons through direct experience. When participants apply what they've learned in real situations requiring cooperation, patience, problem-solving and communication, the learning becomes embodied. Nothing reinforces treatment concepts like natural beauty paired with physical challenge and group cooperation.

The outdoor environment also provides a powerful setting for relationship-building. When people cook together, hike together, set up camp or face difficult terrain as a group, bonds form through shared effort, not forced discussion. These relationships are often the ones that last. Months after treatment, when stress returns and old triggers reappear, people rarely call their counselor. They call the person who stood beside them when they were struggling—their accountability partner, their peer. Your role is to create an environment where those relationships can form and strengthen.

Nature also invites humility. Many patients feel drawn to the outdoors but are not entirely comfortable there. That slight discomfort opens a door. Addiction often involves layers of self-protection, ego, defensiveness and self-involvement. In unfamiliar natural settings, these defenses soften. The person has room to breathe, to try, to fail safely and to grow. The outdoors allows access to parts of the self that may have been closed off for years.

Wilderness therapy programs work best when they combine adventure-based activities with evidence-informed clinical approaches. Multi-day expeditions, hiking, rock climbing, canoeing and other skill-building experiences can be paired with group and individual therapy. The setting becomes a living laboratory for trust, responsibility, resilience and emotional regulation. Engagement is not a problem here; people want to participate. Think about the child who is excited to go fishing at dawn; they are awake long before the alarm. That is the level of intrinsic motivation we are trying to tap into.

Finally, do not outsource this. Develop your program internally, with your own clinical and support staff. Your staff knows your patients and your culture. They are trained to build safe, respectful therapeutic relationships. A generic third-party outdoor provider cannot replicate that. Build a curriculum that grows out of your community, not Joe's Rock Climbing Shop. No offense to Joe.

Measuring Safety: The Intangible Made Tangible

Measuring safety within treatment environments presents unique challenges, for a couple of reasons. Because addictions survive in isolation, people with addictions become practiced at hiding their addiction and deceiving people during the time when they're addicted—so well that the habit is hard to break. Many programs help patients identify this manipulative trait, which then becomes a point of improvement for that patient, but this trait, whether it was learned early in life or developed to protect the addiction, is most likely ingrained in the patient's behavior. During the assessment, they'll know exactly what to say and how to say it so that everything is rosy.

The best detection system is one in which trained staff is the fulcrum, because patient engagement and safe environments are largely intangible. Staff should be trained to recognize signs of safety regularly. (Regularly here means daily.) Your center should initiate daily and weekly meetings where staff members score their observations of the environment and patient engagement based on specific criteria unique to your center, which will provide critical data for continuous improvement in this area. Remember that a good environment can change to a bad one in days—sometimes minutes. This vigilance costs almost nothing and makes a tremendous difference on multiple levels.

There are a few quantitative and qualitative metrics that can provide some insight, such as incident rates, patient satisfaction scores, treatment completion rates and regular focus groups that gather detailed feedback about patients' experiences of safety and support. Use these along with the staff score to come up with a bigger picture of where you're at environmentally.

Lastly, cultural competency represents a crucial component of safety-focused care, recognizing that individuals from different cultural backgrounds may have different needs and expectations regarding safety and support. This includes understanding how multigenerational trauma, discrimination and cultural stigma around mental health and addiction may impact an individual's ability to feel safe in treatment settings. Keep these factors in mind when structuring your center's dynamics.

Section 2: The Framework—"Customized" and Continuous Care

Here's where we get to one of the most significant paradigm shifts in modern addiction recovery: the evolution from standardized treatment protocols to truly "Customized Care." As we established in Chapter 1, addiction is customized to the individual, and therefore recovery programs must also be customized to the individual. This isn't rocket science, but apparently it's more complicated than most treatment centers can handle.

This goes far beyond the familiar concepts of individualized treatment plans or personalized medicine that most centers use as marketing buzzwords while running everyone through identical programs. We're talking about fundamentally reimagining the patient-provider relationship, placing individuals at the center of their own recovery process as active participants in designing and implementing their treatment approach. As we begin this discussion, it should be understood that this presupposes that we are working with a patient who truly wants to get help. If your patient doesn't display this quality, then you must go back to Section 1 and provide an environment where your patient can make the decision to want to change, to want to get help. I'm talking here about the patient that thinks *maybe I've had my last drink— maybe I can do this*.

The Assessment Revolution

"Customized Care" begins with comprehensive assessment processes that explore far more than traditional diagnostic criteria and insurance requirements. Multidimensional evaluation tools should examine personal history, cultural background, learning style, spiritual beliefs, family dynamics, trauma experiences, strengths and aspirations. Most importantly, this assessment must be conducted collaboratively, with patients actively participating in identifying their own needs, preferences and goals rather than simply answering standardized questions designed by committees.

Here's what most centers miss entirely: Patient education during assessment is crucial. Many individuals haven't found success in previous recovery attempts because nobody helped them unlock the specific combination of factors driving their addiction. This requires teaching patients about multiple addiction theories during the assessment process itself, helping them understand that their particular "brand of challenge" likely stems from a complex interaction of neurobiological, psychological, social and environmental factors rather than a single cause.

What we're proposing here is genuinely radical: The treatment profession should work collaboratively with patients to unlock this unique combination. When you have an engaged patient in front of you, and you educate them about the many factors that could contribute to their addiction, such as brain chemistry, trauma history, learned behaviors, family patterns, environmental triggers and spiritual emptiness, you'll see them naturally gravitate toward the elements that resonate with their lived experience. They'll identify what feels true for them and what they think they need to work on.

This creates genuine buy-in on their treatment plan. It's no longer something imposed from outside, but their own understanding of what they need to do to be successful in recovery. Couple this insight with the expertise of trained professionals who can identify additional factors the patient may not recognize, and you can develop a comprehensive treatment plan that might actually move the needle.

Let's be honest about what happens in most treatment centers: It's a chat in front of an expert who asks questions from a predetermined list, checks boxes on a form and lets an algorithm spit out a treatment plan that's virtually identical to what the other three people admitted this week received. Same diagnosis, same program, same expected outcome— which is to say, same disappointing results.

This assembly-line approach fundamentally misunderstands addiction. If addiction is customized to the individual, shaped by their unique biology, history, trauma, relationships and circumstances, then recovery must be equally customized. A collaborative assessment process that educates while it evaluates, and invites participation rather than just extracting information, creates the foundation for treatment that actually addresses each person's specific needs rather than forcing everyone through identical programs designed for hypothetical "average" patients who don't actually exist.

Patients don't have to be passive victims of the healthcare system. With the right technology and mindset, they can become the CEOs of their own health, making informed decisions and taking control of their care.

The practical implementation of "Customized Care" requires sophisticated frameworks for matching individuals to treatment approaches based on their unique characteristics and preferences. Treatment centers must develop assessments that consider personality type, learning style, trauma history, cultural background, family dynamics and personal values. These frameworks help guide the collaborative process of designing treatment plans that resonate with each person's specific needs and circumstances rather than generic programs that treat everyone like interchangeable parts.

Shared Decision-Making Protocols

The most innovative treatment centers should implement shared decision-making protocols that formalize collaborative treatment planning processes. These protocols ensure that patients aren't just consulted about their treatment preferences but are actively involved in weighing different options, understanding potential benefits and risks and making informed decisions about their care through exit strategy.

This approach has been shown to increase treatment engagement, improve adherence to treatment recommendations and enhance overall satisfaction with the recovery process. More importantly, it develops the decision-making skills, personal agency and buy-in that individuals need for long-term recovery success, rather than creating dependence on external direction.

The Continuum Challenge: Actually Connecting Care

As we discussed extensively in Chapter 4, fragmented care and premature discharge create revolving doors rather than lasting recovery. Here's the brutal truth: Most treatment centers talk about continuums of care while operating completely disconnected services that hand people off like hot potatoes the moment their insurance coverage changes.

A true continuum of care creates a seamless thread of treatment that begins when someone decides to seek help and continues throughout their recovery journey, adapting to changing needs while maintaining consistent support and coordination. This isn't about keeping people in treatment forever. It's about maintaining connection and support as they transition through different phases of recovery.

Research consistently shows that individuals who receive coordinated care across multiple treatment levels have significantly better outcomes than those who experience fragmented services. Participation in continuing care programs significantly improves long-term abstinence rates. Yet most centers act like their responsibility ends the moment someone walks out the door.

Technology and Care Coordination

Modern treatment centers should implement patient portal systems that allow individuals to access treatment plans, appointment schedules and educational resources from any location. Mobile applications can provide daily check-ins, medication reminders and direct communication with care teams. Telehealth platforms enable continued therapy sessions even when geographic barriers might otherwise interrupt care.

Predictive analytics can identify patients at high risk for treatment dropout or relapse during transitions. By analyzing patterns in patient data, these systems can flag individuals who may need additional support and automatically trigger enhanced coordination protocols. For example, if the system identifies that a patient has multiple risk factors for early departure from outpatient treatment, it might automatically schedule more frequent check-ins, assign a peer support specialist or arrange for family involvement in the transition process.

Community Partnerships That Actually Work

Successful continuum has a catcher in front of the pitcher. I'm talking about a solid handoff to partnerships with community-based organizations, sober living facilities and outpatient providers. Treatment centers should maintain formal agreements with networks of community partners, establishing clear protocols for referrals, communication and shared care planning. The list of community partners is healthy when a center's outreach personnel are regularly visiting these facilities. These partnerships ensure that patients have immediate access to appropriate services at each level of care without waiting lists or administrative delays that can derail recovery momentum. When they can't do that, it's time to extend the list of partnerships.

Section 3: The Tools—Integrating Multiple Healing Modalities

Here's where most treatment centers completely lose their way. Different aspects of recovery require different tools and approaches, but instead of thoughtful integration, most centers either ignore everything except medication or throw random therapeutic activities at people hoping something sticks. Neither approach works, and both represent fundamental failures to understand what we established in Section 2 about "Customized Care."

Think about it: If the collaborative assessment process reveals that someone's addiction stems from a unique combination of unresolved trauma, dysregulated brain chemistry, learned family patterns, social isolation and spiritual emptiness, you can't address that complexity with a single intervention or even a handful of disconnected therapies. Being diverse in your healing modalities isn't optional. It fits directly into a "Customized Care" approach as a practical necessity.

This section addresses several important therapeutic tools and frameworks that didn't fit neatly into previous discussions, elaborates on approaches we've mentioned briefly and introduces additional modalities that forward-thinking treatment centers should consider integrating into their comprehensive programs.

Dual Diagnosis: The Reality Most Centers Ignore

Here's the thing about dual diagnosis treatment that most centers still don't understand: When someone enters treatment with both mental health and substance use issues, which describes a lot of the people seeking help, you need staff who can address both conditions simultaneously. You can't treat depression on Tuesday and addiction on Thursday and expect them to integrate effectively. Like a DJ who can seamlessly blend two songs, you need to know both tracks and understand how they work together. This requires specialized training and a completely different approach to treatment planning than most centers currently provide.

Medication-Assisted Treatment Done Right

Let's talk about medication-assisted treatment, a recap from Chapter 3 but worth bringing up briefly here. Some people think using medication to treat addiction is like using alcohol to treat alcoholism. But here's what the research actually shows:

For some people, medications like Suboxone or Vivitrol can be game changers when they're part of comprehensive programs. The key word here is "comprehensive." Medication alone is like having a really good foundation for a house but never building the walls or roof, and telling your friends, "I got me a house." When medications are integrated into comprehensive programs that include trauma-informed therapy, family work and psychosocial support, they serve as bridges to comprehensive treatment rather than permanent maintenance solutions. Do the whole program or don't do any of the program.

Nutrition and Physical Wellness: The Foundation Nobody Talks About

Here's something that sounds boring but is absolutely crucial: nutrition and physical wellness. When someone has been using substances for years, their body is basically running on empty. Their brain chemistry is scrambled, their digestive system is compromised and they probably haven't had a decent night's sleep in months. You can't build lasting recovery on a foundation of energy drinks and processed food.

The centers that understand this don't just serve healthy meals; they teach people how to shop, cook and fuel their bodies in ways that support their recovery. They understand that nutrition education is a crucial component of comprehensive care that addresses the physical foundation required for healing, not just an afterthought or something to fill time between therapy sessions.

Additionally, fill your patients' time with physical activities. Outdoors, indoors, do all of it. Go to the gym, *build* a gym, do exercise activities in the hallway. When physical activities are adopted, you help move patients quicker into a healthy state of recovery by moving toxins out of their bodies. Also, patients are at your center to change their lives, and therefore their person must change. Almost any activity is much more engaging than active drug use. "Yeah, I used every day, and I was preparing for an Ironman race at the same time"—said no patient ever!

Spiritual Dimensions

It may surprise some people, but addressing the spiritual dimension of recovery is often crucial for long-term healing. This isn't necessarily about organized religion, though it can include that. It's about meaning, purpose, values and a sense of connection to something larger than the individual self. It may look like traditional faith practices, meditation, time in nature, a personal code of conduct or service to others. The form isn't the point. The point is that humans need purpose to thrive.

There are two key takeaways here.

1. This exploration must be rooted in *their* beliefs and values—not yours.
2. Your role is to create the *environment* where they are free to remember, rediscover or define what feels true to them.

You don't give them a Higher Power. You give them the space to find one. Let's acknowledge something clearly. The 12-step model has spread across the world with measurable success in cultures whose dominant spiritual traditions look nothing like those in the United States. As a Christian myself, I understand how passages like "Thou shalt put no other gods before me" or "I am a jealous God" are often interpreted narrowly. Yet the 12-step program works in communities that call God by entirely different names and sometimes no name at all. It works when someone invokes Jesus, and it works when someone invokes Buddha, Allah, Creator, Spirit or simply the idea of compassion.

So what does that tell us? That the relationship matters more than the label. You don't need to resolve the theology. You just need to be okay with someone finding healing through a conception of the divine that looks different from yours. Your job is not to police belief—your job is to support recovery. Create a safe environment where seeking, questioning, remembering and reconnecting can occur. That's enough.

Family Systems: Healing the Whole Network

Addiction impacts entire family systems. Effective treatment includes family work not as an afterthought, but as core programming. This means helping family members learn to communicate honestly, set boundaries without withdrawing and support recovery without enabling self-destructive patterns. When done well, this work strengthens the support system long past discharge. (See Chapter 5 for deeper application.)

Peer Support: Where the Magic Really Happens

There is something uniquely powerful about connecting with someone who has walked the same path as you. Peer Recovery Support Specialists bring lived experience alongside training, and that combination bridges the gap between clinical insight and real-world survival. The best treatment centers integrate peer support from intake through long-term follow-up. Recovery is sustained in relationships, and peers often provide the hope and accountability that formal therapy alone cannot.

Mindfulness or Meditation: Advanced Neuroscience Integration

Dr. Dispenza's work on meditation and neural pathway transformation provides another crucial component of integrated treatment approaches, though his methods require careful adaptation for clinical settings. Unlike traditional mindfulness practices that focus on present-moment awareness, Dr. Dispenza's approach emphasizes intentional meditation practices designed specifically to rewire neural pathways and create new patterns of thinking, feeling and behaving.[87]

The implementation involves teaching individuals to become acutely aware of their unconscious thoughts, behaviors and emotions, not just to observe them, but to consciously interrupt old patterns and install new ones. Through specific meditation techniques, individuals learn to disassociate from past emotional states and literally rehearse new ways of thinking and feeling during structured practice sessions.

The meditation practices differ significantly from traditional mindfulness techniques. Rather than simply observing thoughts and feelings, individuals learn to actively generate new emotional states and rehearse new behavioral patterns during meditation. This includes feeling the emotions associated with their future recovered self and making decisions from this elevated state rather than from past conditioning.

However, integration of these approaches into clinical addiction treatment programs requires bringing in a Neuro-ChangeSolutions Consultant with careful consideration, program adaptation and consultation to ensure the program is right for your patient population.

HeartMath and heart-brain coherence training using biofeedback technology teaches individuals to achieve synchronization between heart rhythms and brain waves through specialized training and breathing techniques. This innovative approach helps patients develop real-time awareness of their nervous system states and learn to shift from stress to calm quickly, a skill that proves invaluable in managing triggers and cravings. Patients use biofeedback devices during meditation sessions, therapy appointments and throughout daily life to build coherence between their cardiovascular and nervous systems. Research demonstrates that individuals who achieve heart-brain coherence show significantly improved stress tolerance, emotional stability and overall treatment engagement. [88]

Virtual Reality and Technology Integration

Technology isn't just changing how we communicate or work; it's revolutionizing how we heal. Beyond basic applications, a few treatment centers are now using virtual reality systems that can create immersive experiences allowing individuals to practice new behaviors, confront triggers in safe environments and literally see themselves in their future recovered identity.

Some treatment centers have developed VR programs that combine exposure therapy for addiction triggers with positive visualization experiences that reinforce recovery identity and goals. Biofeedback systems literally teach your nervous system how to regulate itself, mobile apps put meditation teachers in your pocket and wearable devices provide real-time feedback about stress levels. It's like having a personal wellness coach that never sleeps.

Success in the whole treatment process can't be measured solely by counting sober days, though that certainly matters. Quality of life, relationship health, sense of purpose, emotional stability and overall life satisfaction provide more meaningful measures of transformation.

Here's something that might change how you think about recovery conversations: Instead of leading every interaction with someone in recovery by asking "How many days sober are you?"—as if that's the most important question—try asking "What has your sobriety meant to you?" or "How has your life changed since your recovery began?" These questions focus on what we really want to know: the quality and meaning of the transformation, not just its duration. They also serve to reinforce the success had by the recovering addict. As they regale you with stories of how wonderful their life has become and how freeing sobriety is, they leave you that day feeling better about themselves, their efforts and the trajectory of their new life. So, for their sake, ask the right questions.

Section 4: The System—Organizational Architecture for Transformation

We're not talking about tweaking existing treatment programs or adding new services to the same broken foundation. We're discussing completely rebuilding how addiction treatment organizations operate from the ground up. It's the difference between renovating a house and tearing it down to build something entirely new—the old foundation simply won't support what we're trying to create.

Think about this: We're dealing with a condition that kills more people annually than gun violence and car accidents combined. Yet we're running treatment systems with organizational structures that would make a 1970s manufacturing plant look progressive. Something must change, and it shouldn't be small adjustments around the edges.

Flipping the Traditional Hierarchy

The staffing model in transformative treatment centers flips traditional hierarchies completely. Instead of credentialed experts at the top dictating to everyone else what recovery should look like, collaborative teams honor different types of expertise. The person with a PhD in psychology works alongside someone whose PhD comes from the school of hard knocks, and both perspectives are valued equally.

These centers prioritize hiring people with lived experience because credibility in addiction treatment often comes from having walked the walk, not just memorizing the research. When someone in early recovery sees staff members who have successfully navigated the same journey, it provides hope and practical wisdom that can't be taught in any graduate program.

But this isn't about hiring people just because they're in recovery. It's about finding individuals who combine lived experience with the ability to help others, who possess both the emotional stability to handle challenging situations and the professional skills necessary to work in healthcare settings. The combination of personal experience and professional competence creates incredibly powerful therapeutic relationships.

I want to add something I've learned firsthand. I've worked in many industries, hired all kinds of people and managed teams in very different environments. Through that experience, I've noticed something important: Individuals in active recovery who are genuinely working their program have usually done more honest self-examination than most people will do in a lifetime.

It's difficult to find someone outside of recovery who will look you in the eye and say, "I'm a work in progress. If there's something I need to improve, tell me and I'll get to work on it." The truth is, that level of humility and willingness to grow is rare. Far more often, in other industries, I've seen the opposite—people who believe that once they have a credential, they're done learning. Any suggestion for improvement feels like a threat, not an opportunity.

By contrast, many people in recovery are actively involved in ongoing personal growth. They've identified their patterns, owned their mistakes and learned how to confront themselves honestly. That mindset, when genuine, makes for exceptional employees, teammates and leaders.

The same can be true for individuals returning from incarceration who have done real rehabilitation work. When someone has confronted themselves deeply, rebuilt their identity and chosen a different path, they often bring the traits of accountability, resilience, loyalty and work ethic that are hard to teach. I'm grateful to work in a field where we can hire and support people who have rebuilt their lives and are committed to growth. That's what citizenship looks like.

Physical Spaces That Actually Heal

Walk into a transformative treatment center and you immediately notice it doesn't feel like a medical facility designed by someone who confused "sterile" with "healing." Natural lighting floods comfortable gathering spaces. Private nooks invite reflection and contemplation. Outdoor areas encourage connection with nature. Every design choice asks: Does this support healing or hinder it?

Here's an idea for you: Add a sensory room to your space. A sensory room is a curated, specifically built and designed environment that provides graded sensory input to promote calm and relaxation. This space creates an environment where patients can step away from other stimulants and practice the art of self-regulation. There are times in recovery, just like in life, when everything gets too heavy and a personal reset is necessary. Sensory rooms provide that space for overwhelmed patients.

Even basic considerations matter—like ensuring staff have the right tools to do their jobs. Functional computers and printers, comfortable break rooms with good coffee and vacation time that they must take throughout the year make the difference between what is healthy and what is not. When staff feel supported and valued, they're better able to create supportive environments for the people they serve.

Technology in Service of Transformation

Technology integration isn't about digitizing old processes to improve efficiency; it's about using innovation to enhance healing in ways that were never possible before. Consider the use of biofeedback systems that teach individuals to regulate their nervous systems in real time. Consider customizing a mobile app that will help you track recovery and provide ongoing support and connection that extends far beyond treatment walls.

Measuring What Actually Matters

There are few centers that measure success completely differently from traditional programs. I invite you to become one of them. Abstinence and program completion are metrics that matter because they measure personal empowerment, life satisfaction, relationship quality and sense of purpose. Prioritizing these statistics will help you understand that true recovery isn't just about stopping substance use—it's about creating a life so compelling that addiction becomes irrelevant. Remember, sobriety is not recovery.

Long-term follow-up becomes essential for understanding real outcomes. Checking in at intervals of 30, 60 and 90 days and on months six, 12, 18, 24, 36, 48 and 60 provides data that is much more meaningful than success measures at 30 days post-completion. As I've said, 30-day post-completion rates are designed primarily to satisfy regulators and insurance companies rather than measure actual transformation.

Community Integration: Recovery Happens in Community

Community partnerships are crucial because lasting recovery requires support extending far beyond the treatment center. These centers develop relationships with local organizations, businesses, schools and community groups, understanding that recovery happens in community, not in isolation.

Employment assistance, housing support, educational opportunities and ongoing social connections all contribute to sustainable recovery outcomes. Treatment centers should actively help people rebuild their place in the community rather than just preparing them to leave treatment. Note that the staff member who has the most effective impact in this area is the case manager, and the most effective case manager-patient relationships extend well beyond the prescribed course of treatment.

Alumni Programs: The Virtuous Cycle

Alumni programs create ongoing communities of support lasting for years after formal treatment ends. If you don't have an alumni program, start one today. Regular social activities, educational opportunities, mentorship programs and service opportunities allow people in recovery to give back to others beginning their journey.

This creates a virtuous cycle of healing and support where those who have found recovery become resources and inspiration for those still seeking it. Alumni programs also provide treatment centers with ongoing feedback about long-term outcomes and opportunities for continuous program improvement. Other ideas include allowing the alumni to organize themselves into an advisory board or asking them to plan and run the calendar and sponsor family outings and activities. You, the treatment center, should be as supportive of their plans as possible.

Section 5: Financial Sustainability and Creative Funding Solutions

Let's address the elephant in the room. It's the thing most treatment administrators spend more time worrying about than actually helping people: money.

How do you fund the myriad treatment ideas mentioned in this book when they cost more up front than the cookie-cutter programs that insurance companies prefer to reimburse? Here's the uncomfortable truth: You don't—at least not with the profit you made last year.

The Hard Decisions: Program Before Profits

Here's where we separate organizations that are truly committed to transformation from those that just want to sound innovative in their marketing. If you want real change, you have to be willing to make hard decisions that put program effectiveness before profit margins.

What I'm about to say is the most radical idea in this entire book:

Sometimes helping people requires sacrificing profit.

There are moments when doing what is best for the patient will not be what is best for the company's bottom line. And I understand that this is where some people will check out. But I didn't spend all this time outlining what's broken in the treatment industry just to end with "Good luck—hope the numbers work out."

If you've read this far, it's because you already know something is broken in your own system. You've been nodding along, thinking, *Yes, that's true. Yes, that needs to change. Yes, we can do better.* The natural next question is: So what do we do now?

For me, the answer came years ago:

I chose effectiveness over profit.

I chose outcomes over comfort.

130

I chose patients over margins.

We made operational decisions that cost money, sometimes a significant amount, because they created better care, better culture, better long-term recovery and better human outcomes. And it was worth it. Now, if you're not ready to commit to that fully, that's okay—but let me offer you a few starting points.

Nonprofit Strategies and Grant Funding

Treatment centers committed to comprehensive, patient-centered care should seriously consider nonprofit status if they haven't already. I'm suggesting that we use the nonprofit model for its original purpose: to serve the community.

You don't have to reinvent your operations. Keep your existing structure, staffing and overhead. Transitioning to nonprofit status simply allows you to redirect the money you would have paid in taxes toward the kinds of programming that truly improve outcomes. Yes, there are pros and cons here, but it is an option worth genuine consideration.

Nonprofit status also opens doors that are closed to for-profit facilities: foundation grants, federal and state funding streams, donor partnerships and corporate social responsibility initiatives. Many companies—healthcare systems, technology firms and local employers—are looking for meaningful ways to address the addiction crisis affecting their own workforce and communities. When you become a nonprofit, you become eligible for that support.

You already have a marketing department. Redirect that same budget and staffing into development and fundraising. The outlay stays the same, but now the work directly fuels your mission rather than just your census.

This is how you return to the reason you entered this field in the first place: to build a treatment center that actually helps people get healthy. Not just on paper, not just in metrics, but in real life.

Value-Based Care: Paying for Outcomes

Some centers have moved beyond traditional fee-for-service approaches to value-based contracts that pay for outcomes rather than services. Instead of getting paid for bed days or therapy sessions, these centers get rewarded for keeping people in recovery long-term. Imagine that—a healthcare system that actually pays providers for keeping people healthy. Structure this smartly and you should be making more for the healthy patient because insurance pays less for the unhealthy patient.

These arrangements require sophisticated outcome-tracking systems and the willingness to put your money where your mouth is regarding treatment effectiveness. They also create genuine alignment between financial incentives and patient well-being, which should be implied but apparently isn't in most healthcare settings.

Creative Revenue Diversification

Training and consultation services can generate revenue while spreading effective practices to other centers. Organizations that develop innovative approaches can offer training programs, consultation services and licensing opportunities to other treatment providers interested in implementing similar models.

Alumni and family programs can be partially fee-supported for individuals who can afford to contribute, creating sustainable funding for ongoing services while maintaining sliding-scale access for those who cannot pay.

Research partnerships with universities can provide funding for innovative program evaluation while contributing to the broader evidence base for effective treatment approaches. Academic partnerships also provide access to graduate student research assistance and faculty expertise that can enhance program development.

Sliding Scale and Scholarship Programs

Treatment centers committed to transformation should establish robust sliding fee scales and scholarship programs ensuring that financial barriers don't prevent access to comprehensive care. This isn't charity—it's good business practice that builds community support and demonstrates genuine commitment to mission over profit.

Scholarship programs can be funded through alumni donations, community fundraising events, corporate sponsorships and percentage allocations from full-pay clients. Many successful centers find that their scholarship programs become powerful marketing tools that demonstrate their values while generating community support. That could allow you to minimize your marketing budget, which increases your profit, therefore allowing you to add more to your treatment program.

Financial Transparency and Accountability

Centers pursuing innovative funding approaches should implement transparent financial reporting that demonstrates how funds are used to improve patient outcomes rather than enrich administrators. This transparency builds trust with donors, partners and regulatory agencies while ensuring accountability for innovative program investments.

Conclusion: The Blueprint for Transformation

The transformation of addiction treatment from symptom management to lasting recovery creation is not just possible, it's already happening in scattered locations across the country. These pioneering facilities prove that when we move beyond outdated models and embrace comprehensive, individualized approaches addressing the whole person, extraordinary outcomes become achievable rather than accidental.

The areas outlined in this chapter—foundational safety and connection, "Customized" continuous care frameworks, integrated healing modalities, transformative organizational systems and creative financial sustainability—represent a comprehensive blueprint for reimagining addiction treatment. These aren't theoretical concepts developed in academic committee meetings but practical, evidence-based approaches being implemented successfully in real-world settings by people who decided that the status quo kills too many people to defend. You don't have to do all of them; pick the ones that fit your center best and run with them.

The evidence is unambiguous and frankly embarrassing for those still defending traditional approaches. Individuals receiving coordinated, comprehensive, individualized care have significantly better outcomes than those receiving fragmented, standardized services. They stay in treatment longer, achieve recovery at higher rates, maintain recovery over the long term and report higher levels of life satisfaction, stronger relationships and greater sense of purpose. In other words, they use words like "lifelong recovery" instead of "program completion."

The transformation requires courage. Courage to abandon approaches that have failed spectacularly in favor of those that succeed, courage to invest in comprehensive care despite significant up-front costs and courage to trust in human potential and resilience even when individuals have experienced repeated treatment failures. It also requires admitting that much of what we've been doing for decades has been more about making providers feel better than actually helping patients get better.

But transformation also requires practical action that goes beyond good intentions and inspiring mission statements. Treatment providers must invest in staff training, technology infrastructure and organizational culture change. Administrators must measure success differently and advocate for policy changes supporting innovative approaches rather than just complaining about insurance companies. Policymakers must create regulatory frameworks that encourage rather than inhibit innovation and effectiveness.

The addiction crisis demands complete reimagining of treatment and recovery approaches. The solutions exist, the evidence is clear and the technology is available to support these approaches. What's untapped is the collective will to implement these solutions at scale and create a treatment system that truly serves the people it claims to help, rather than the financial interests of those who profit from their continued suffering.

The future of addiction treatment isn't about finding one perfect approach for everyone. That unicorn doesn't exist, and pursuing it wastes time while people die. It's about developing sophisticated methods to help each person find the unique combination of approaches that works for them specifically. This personalized, integrative, "Customized" approach represents the cutting edge of addiction treatment, offering hope for individuals who haven't responded to traditional approaches and providing a roadmap for treatment systems that honor the complexity and uniqueness of human experience rather than treating people like interchangeable parts in an assembly line.

The transformation of addiction treatment isn't just a clinical imperative. It's a moral imperative that reflects our fundamental values about human worth and potential. Every day we delay implementing these proven approaches, people continue suffering and dying from a condition that is treatable. All we need is the courage to treat it comprehensively and the wisdom to abandon approaches that don't work.

The time for incremental change, pilot programs and cautious experimentation has passed. The addiction crisis demands bold action, innovative thinking and the willingness to completely rebuild systems that have failed. The blueprint exists. The question isn't whether these approaches work; the question is whether we have the courage and commitment necessary to implement them before more people die waiting for us to figure out what we already know.

The time for transformation is now. The only question remaining is whether you're ready to be part of the solution or whether you'll continue defending a system that everyone knows doesn't work.

The solutions outlined in this chapter build on everything we've established throughout this book. From the individualized approaches of Chapter 1 to the equity principles of Chapter 6, we have the knowledge and tools necessary for transformation. What we need now is the collective will to implement them and the courage to abandon approaches that have failed in favor of those that succeed. The future of addiction treatment, and the lives of millions of people, depend on our willingness to act on what we already know.

8

To the Reader—A Guide for Moving Forward

Three people sit in different cities, each holding a copy of this book, each having reached the final chapter with vastly different emotions.

In Portland, Rachel closes the book and stares at the wall. With two failed rehab attempts behind her, she's been shuttled between programs that treated her trauma as irrelevant and her need for longer-term care as insurance fraud. But something in these pages has shifted her perspective. For the first time, she isn't blaming herself for the failures. The system is broken, not her.

In Atlanta, Michael sets the book down and rubs his temples. His daughter Emma has been in and out of treatment for three years. He'd hoped to find the magic answer, the perfect program. Instead, he'd found a devastating indictment of everything they'd tried. But the book gave him something more valuable: understanding. Emma's addiction isn't a moral failing; it is a complex response requiring comprehensive, individualized care.

In Chicago, Dr. Jennifer Martinez closes her laptop. As a treatment center clinical director, she'd felt every criticism like a personal attack. But as her anger cools, honesty creeps in.

Their success rates were abysmal. They discharged people based on insurance timelines rather than clinical readiness. The book held up a mirror, and she didn't like what she saw. But she now feels determination. If the system is broken, she is in a position to help fix it.

I don't know who you are, but I have a pretty good idea why you're reading this book. Maybe you're someone struggling with addiction, desperately searching for answers that actually make sense. Maybe you're a family member watching someone you love destroy themselves while the system fails them repeatedly. Or maybe you're a treatment professional who either loves what we've written because it validates what you've been seeing, or is furious because we've challenged everything you've been taught to believe.

Whoever you are, this chapter is for you. Not as a patient, a client or a case study, but as a human being deserving of honest, practical guidance based on everything we've learned about what actually works in recovery.

If You're Someone Struggling with Addiction

First, let me say something that the treatment industry often gets wrong: You are not broken. You are not diseased. You are not powerless. You are a human being who has been using substances to solve problems that substances can't actually solve, and now you've created a bigger problem. But any problem can be solved when you have the right tools and the right support.

The confusion you feel when choosing treatment options isn't a character flaw. It's a rational response to a field that can't agree on what addiction is, let alone how to treat it effectively. Your repeated treatment failures likely reflect inadequate care, not personal deficiency.

The most important thing you need to understand is that recovery is not about finding the perfect program. It's about finding the right combination of approaches that work for you. The treatment center that saved your friend's life might be completely wrong for your situation. The approach that failed you last time might work perfectly when combined with something different. You are unique, and your recovery needs to be unique too.

What to Look for in Treatment

Here's what to look for in any treatment approach: Does it treat you like a whole person, or just like a brain that needs fixing? Does it address the trauma, pain and circumstances that led to your addiction, or does it just focus on stopping the substance use? Does it help you build a life worth living, or does it just teach you how to white-knuckle through cravings?

Most importantly, does it respect your intelligence and involve you in decisions about your own care? You should be an active participant in designing your recovery, not a passive recipient of other people's solutions. If a program tells you to "just trust the process" without explaining what the process is or why it should work for you, keep looking.

Demand programs that address trauma, not just symptoms. If a program doesn't conduct comprehensive trauma assessments or offer trauma-informed care, walk away. The majority of people with addiction have significant trauma histories. Treating addiction without addressing underlying trauma is like treating a broken bone without setting it first.

Insist on individualized treatment plans, not cookie-cutter approaches. Your treatment plan should address your specific trauma history, mental health conditions, family dynamics and social circumstances. It should evolve as you progress, not follow predetermined timelines based on insurance coverage.

Seek programs that integrate evidence-based approaches with holistic care. The most effective treatment combines proven therapeutic modalities, cognitive behavioral therapy, dialectical behavior therapy and EMDR for trauma with complementary approaches addressing the whole person. Beware of programs relying exclusively on any single approach or even two approaches.

Demand adequate length of treatment based on clinical need, not insurance timelines. Your recovery timeline is not anyone else's recovery timeline. Don't let insurance companies, treatment centers or even well-meaning family members pressure you into believing that 30 days, 90 days or any other arbitrary number represents "enough" treatment. Your brain didn't get addicted on a schedule, and it won't recover on one either. Healing takes as long as it takes. Remember, you got yourself into this mess over the past 10, 20, 30 years. Don't think that someone is going to wave a magic wand in your face and fix you in 30 days.

Developing Recovery Attributes

The virtues that will serve you most in recovery are brutally simple but incredibly powerful. Be honest, not just about your substance use, but about your feelings, your fears, your dreams and your pain. The lies we tell ourselves are often more dangerous than the substances we use. Demonstrate integrity; make your actions match your values, even when it's difficult. This means showing up when you say you will, following through on commitments and being the same person in private that you are in public. Take ownership of your choices, your recovery and your life without falling into the trap of shame or blame.

Here's something crucial: Being open about your struggles isn't a sign of weakness; it's a sign of strength. Addiction thrives in secrecy and isolation. Generally, recovery happens in connection and community. You don't have to share your deepest secrets with everyone, but you need at least a few people who know the real you and support your recovery anyway.

Find approaches that make sense to you. If the spiritual aspects of 12-step programs don't resonate with you, that doesn't mean you're doing recovery wrong; it means you need a different approach. If traditional therapy feels too slow, explore action-oriented approaches. If sitting in rooms talking about problems makes you want to use, try activities that build your body and spirit alongside your mind.

Pay attention to your body, not just your brain. Addiction affects everything—your nutrition, your sleep, your physical fitness, your stress levels. You can't build lasting recovery on a foundation of energy drinks and fast food. Movement, nutrition, sleep and stress management aren't optional; they're fundamental.

One more thing to keep in mind: Your brain is saturated with chemicals from the last several years of using, and your dopamine levels are all out of whack. (That's the technical term, right?) Generally, you are physically unable to make your best decisions while in this state. You may have to rely on someone, trust someone, to help you make better decisions. Pick a loved one, a friend, someone who resonates with you. Do research with them, work together, seek their advice at least for a little while.

Most importantly, remember that recovery is not about returning to who you were before addiction; it's about becoming who you're meant to be. The person you are in recovery should be better, stronger, more authentic and more alive than the person you were before you ever used substances. Recovery isn't about going backward; it's about going forward into a life you've never lived before.

If You're a Family Member or Loved One

Watching someone you love struggle with addiction is one

of the most helpless, frustrating and heartbreaking experiences a person can endure. You've probably tried everything: pleading, threatening, bribing, enabling, cutting them off and bringing them back. You've researched treatment centers, attended family meetings and maybe even gone to AA meetings yourself. And yet here you are, still searching for answers.

The first thing you need to understand is that you cannot fix another person's addiction, no matter how much you love them. This isn't a failure on your part—it's the nature of addiction itself. The person you love has to want recovery for themselves, and they have to do the work of recovery themselves. Your job is not to cure them; your job is to stop enabling their addiction while remaining available to support their recovery.

Setting Healthy Boundaries

Learning the difference between helping and enabling is crucial. Helping supports their recovery; enabling supports their addiction. Paying for treatment is helping. Paying their rent so they can spend their money on drugs is enabling. Driving them to therapy appointments is helping. Calling in sick to their job because they're too hungover to work is enabling. The distinction isn't always clear, but here's a good rule of thumb: If what you're doing allows them to avoid the natural consequences of their addiction, it's probably enabling.

Set financial boundaries by refusing to provide money that could be used for substances, but consider paying directly for treatment, therapy or basic necessities. Don't bail them out of legal consequences, but support their access to quality representation. Refuse to lie or cover for them, but don't shame them publicly.

Supporting Evidence-Based Treatment

When you're evaluating treatment options, remember everything we've discussed in this book. Look for programs that treat the whole person, not just the addiction. Ask about trauma-informed care, family involvement and long-term support systems. Be skeptical of programs that promise quick fixes or that seem more interested in your insurance coverage than your loved one's specific needs.

Use knowledge from this book to advocate for comprehensive, trauma-informed care addressing underlying issues rather than just managing symptoms. Research treatment options thoroughly. Ask about their approach to trauma, success rates with long-term follow-up, integration of evidence-based therapies and philosophy about treatment length.

Support longer-term treatment even when insurance coverage ends. The 30-day model fails because it's based on financial convenience, not clinical need.

Taking Care of Yourself

Prepare yourself for the long haul. Addiction recovery is rarely a straight line from active addiction to permanent sobriety. There may be relapses, false starts and setbacks. This doesn't mean treatment doesn't work or that your loved one is hopeless—it means recovery is a process, not an event. Each attempt at recovery, even if it doesn't "stick," can teach valuable lessons and build important skills. In some cases, you can play a role. Help your loved one learn the lessons from their past relapses. Sometimes, they don't see the mistakes others see. Play the "what worked and what didn't" game. What habits or behaviors do they demonstrate when they're sober? What was the trigger that caused them to relapse? What should they do differently next time?

Take care of yourself throughout this process. You can't

pour from an empty cup, and you can't support someone else's recovery if you're falling apart yourself. This might mean therapy for yourself, support groups for families, setting boundaries that protect your own well-being or simply making time for activities that bring you joy and peace.

Seek your own therapy with someone who understands addiction and family dynamics. Join evidence-based support groups for families. Practice self-care consistently and maintain your own relationships, interests and goals even when your loved one is struggling.

Remember that recovery changes everyone in the family, not just the person with the addiction. Support your loved one's recovery efforts without making your well-being dependent on their success. Your love matters, but it's not enough to cure addiction. Your support is valuable, but it's not responsible for their recovery.

If You're an Industry Professional

Some of you are reading this book and nodding your heads, thinking, *Finally, someone is saying what I've been thinking for years.* Others are probably furious that I've had the audacity to challenge approaches you've been taught to see as sacred. To both groups, I say this: Good. I'm glad you're having a strong reaction, because that means you're paying attention.

The moral injury you feel when you are forced to discharge someone you know isn't ready, when you are required to use approaches you know are inadequate, when you are pressured to prioritize billing over healing, is a sign your conscience is intact. Listen to it.

If you're in the first group—if you've been seeing the problems we've described and feeling frustrated by a system that seems designed to fail the people it's supposed to help— then you know what you need to do. Take what resonates with you from this book and start implementing it. Push for changes in your organization. Advocate for approaches that actually work, even if they're not what you've always done. The recovery numbers across the country aren't lying. If you are always doing what you've always done and are constantly hitting weak-tea numbers, then you might be part of the problem, not the solution.

If you're in the second group—if you're convinced that we're wrong, that the approaches we've criticized are actually effective—then I challenge you to do something: Prove us wrong with data, not tradition. Show us the long-term recovery rates from your programs. Demonstrate that 30-day treatments create lasting change. Provide evidence that abstinence-only approaches work better than comprehensive, trauma-informed care.

Embrace Evidence Over Tradition

The question isn't whether you're a good person with good intentions. I believe most people in this field are exactly that. The question is whether you're willing to abandon approaches that don't work in favor of approaches that do, even if it means admitting that much of what you've been taught and practiced has been ineffective.

Abandon the "this is how we've always done it" mentality. Tradition is not evidence. Commit to staying current with addiction research. Question every intervention you use: What's the evidence? How do we measure effectiveness?

This means embracing trauma-informed care as the standard, not the exception. It means extending treatment timelines to match brain healing rather than insurance authorizations. It means involving families in meaningful ways rather than treating addiction as an individual pathology. It means measuring success by life transformation, not just program completion.

Most importantly, it means putting the people you serve at

the center of their own recovery process rather than making them passive recipients of your expertise. The days of "we know what's best for you" medicine are ending, and addiction treatment needs to catch up with the rest of healthcare in embracing collaborative, patient-centered approaches.

The Call to Action

You have a choice to make. You can continue doing what you've always done and getting the results you've always gotten—or you can be part of the revolution that transforms addiction treatment from a system that manages symptoms to one that creates lasting recovery. The people walking through your doors deserve nothing less than your best effort to provide them with approaches that actually work.

You have the opportunity to be part of something revolutionary—the transformation of a broken system into one that actually serves the people it claims to help. The people seeking your help deserve your commitment to excellence, evidence and genuine healing.

The Path Forward

Rachel, Michael and Dr. Martinez represent millions whose lives have been touched by addiction and the broken system that claims to treat it. Their stories continue beyond this book, shaped by the choices they make in response to what they've learned.

Transformation isn't a fairy tale ending. It's a realistic possibility if we refuse to accept inadequate care as inevitable. The transformation of addiction treatment won't be an overnight overhaul. It requires individuals making different choices, one decision at a time.

Addiction is one of the most misunderstood, poorly treated and unnecessarily devastating problems in our society.

But it doesn't have to be. We have the knowledge, the tools and the technology to create recovery systems that actually work. What we need now is the courage to implement them.

To those struggling with addiction: You deserve comprehensive care that addresses your whole person, not just your substance use. Don't settle for programs that treat you like a diagnosis rather than a human being.

To families: You deserve honesty about what works and what doesn't, not false promises designed to separate you from your money during your most vulnerable moments.

To professionals: You have the power to change lives and transform communities. Use it wisely.

The revolution in addiction treatment isn't coming—it's here, in these pages, in your hands, in the decisions you make after closing this book. It starts with refusing to accept failure as inevitable, inadequate care as sufficient or profit as more important than healing.

What will you choose?

Acknowledgments

This book is dedicated to two communities who have profoundly shaped both this work and my life.

To the remarkable staff I have the privilege to work alongside each day: Your unwavering commitment to excellence and your relentless pursuit of innovative improvement inspire me beyond measure. You don't simply show up—you bring passion, creativity and a shared vision for what we can accomplish together. This book exists because of the foundation you help build every single day.

And to the brotherhood at Beacon Treatment Center: Your courage to change, to heal and to grow in the face of extraordinary challenges reminds me daily of the strength of the human spirit. You are not merely changing your own lives —you are transforming the lives of those around you, creating ripples of hope that extend far beyond what you may ever know. Your dedication to recovery and to one another inspires me in every moment, and it is an honor to witness your journey.

To both groups: Thank you for teaching me that true transformation happens in community, through compassion and with an unwavering belief in what's possible.

Bibliography

[1] Sinha, Rajita. "New Findings on Biological Factors Predicting Addiction Relapse Vulnerability." *Current Psychiatry Reports* 13, no. 5 (2011): 398-405. doi:10.1007/s11920-011-0224-0.

[2] Maté, Gabor. *In the Realm of Hungry Ghosts: Close Encounters with Addiction.* Berkeley, CA: North Atlantic Books, 2008.

[3] Broekhof, Rosalie, Hans M. Nordahl, Lars Tanum, and Sara G. Selvik. "Adverse Childhood Experiences and Their Association with Substance Use Disorders in Adulthood: A General Population Study (Young-HUNT)." *Addictive Behaviors Reports* 17 (2023): 100488. doi:10.1016/j.abrep.2023.100488.

[4] Volkow, Nora D., George F. Koob, and Thomas A. McLellan. "Neurobiologic Advances from the Brain Disease Model of Addiction." *The New England Journal of Medicine* 374, no. 4 (2016): 363-371; 374. doi: 10.1056/NEJMra1511480.

[5] Lewis, Marc. *The Biology of Desire: Why Addiction Is Not a Disease.* New York: PublicAffairs, 2015.

[6] Ross, Tom. "Recovery & Treatment of Sexual Addiction: An Interview with Dr. Patrick Carnes." *Open Access Journal of Addiction and Psychology* 4, no. 4 (2022).

[7] Fairbairn, Catharine E., Daniel A. Briley, Dahyeon Kang, R. Chris Fraley, Benjamin L. Hankin, and Talia Ariss. "A Meta-Analysis of Longitudinal Associations between Substance Use and Interpersonal Attachment Security." *Psychological Bulletin* 144, no. 5 (2018): 532-555. doi: 10.1037/bul0000141.

[8] Flores, Philip J. *Addiction as an Attachment Disorder.* 2nd ed. Lanham, MD: Rowman & Littlefield, 2011.

[9] Hari, Johann. "Johann Hari: 'The Opposite of Addiction Isn't Sobriety – It's Connection.'" *The Guardian,* April 12, 2016. https://www.theguardian.com/books/2016/apr/12/johann-hari-chasing-the-scream-war-on-drugs.

[10] Schindler, Andreas (2019). "Attachment and substance use disorders—Theoretical models, empirical evidence, and implications for treatment." *Frontiers in Psychiatry,* 10, 727. doi: 10.3389/fpsyt.2019.00727.

[11] W., Bill. *Alcoholics Anonymous: The Story of How Many Thousands of Men and Women Have Recovered from Alcoholism.* New York: Alcoholics Anonymous World Services, 2002.

[12] Alcoholics Anonymous World Services. "AA History." Alcoholics Anonymous. Accessed October 27, 2025. https://www.aa.org/aa-history.

Bibliography

[13] Dodes, Lance, and Zachary Dodes. *The Sober Truth: Debunking the Bad Science Behind 12-Step Programs and the Rehab Industry.* Boston: Beacon Press, 2014.

[14] Donovan, D. M. (2013). "12-Step interventions and mutual support programs for substance use disorders." *The Journal of Clinical Psychology,* 69(11), 1187-1195. doi: 10.1002/jclp.22079.

[15] Dodes, L., and Z. Dodes (2014). *The Sober Truth.*

[16] Kelly, John F., Alexandra Abry, Marica Ferri, and Keith Humphreys. "Alcoholics Anonymous and 12-Step Facilitation Treatments for Alcohol Use Disorder: A Distillation of a 2020 Cochrane Review for Clinicians and Policy Makers." *Alcohol and Alcoholism* 55, no. 6 (2020): 641-51. doi: 10.1093/alcalc/agaa050.

[17] Lewis, M. (2015). *The Biology of Desire.*

[18] W., Bill (2002). *Alcoholics Anonymous.*

[19] W., Bill (2002). *Alcoholics Anonymous.*

[20] "Opioid Crisis: Addiction, Overprescription, and Insufficient Primary Prevention." *The Lancet Regional Health - Americas* 23 (July 2023): 100557. doi: 10.1016/j.lana.2023.100557.

[21] Chacko, Kesiya. "Addiction Treatment Market Size to Hit USD 16.22 Billion by 2034." *Precedence Research,* July 15, 2025. https://www.precedenceresearch.com/addiction-treatment-market.

[22] "Drugs, Brains, and Behavior: The Science of Addiction - Treatment and Recovery." *National Institutes of Health,* July 2020. https://nida.nih.gov/publications/drugs-brains-behavior-science-addiction/treatment-recovery.

[23] "With Sobering Science, Doctor Debunks 12-Step Recovery." *NPR,* March 23, 2014. https://www.npr.org/2014/03/23/291405829/with-sobering-science-doctor-debunks-12-step-recovery.

[24] Kandasamy, Arun, and Jayakrishnan Menon. "Relapse Prevention." *Indian Journal of Psychiatry* 60, no. 8 (2018): 473. doi: 10.4103/psychiatry.indianjpsychiatry_36_18.

[25] "How Much Does It Cost to Go to Rehab?" *American Addiction Centers.* Accessed October 27, 2025. https://americanaddictioncenters.org/rehab-guide/rehab-cost.

[26] Kelly, John F., Alexandra Abry, Marica Ferri, and Keith Humphreys. "Alcoholics Anonymous and 12-Step Facilitation Treatments for Alcohol Use Disorder: A Distillation of a 2020 Cochrane Review for Clinicians and Policy Makers." *Alcohol and Alcoholism* 55, no. 6 (2020): 641-51. doi: 10.1093/alcalc/agaa050.

[27] "How Purdue Pharma and the Sackler Family Perpetrated the Opioid Crisis." *Addiction Center.* Accessed October 27, 2025. https://www.addictioncenter.com/community/how-purdue-pharma-sackler-family-perpetrated-opioid-crisis/.

[28] "Opioid Overdose: Understanding the Epidemic." *Centers for Disease Control and Prevention.* March 6, 2024. https://www.cdc.gov/drugoverdose/epidemic/index.html.

Bibliography

[29] Joseph, Andrew. "Richard Sackler, Member of Family Behind OxyContin, Was Granted Patent for Addiction Treatment." *STAT News*, September 7, 2018. https://www.statnews.com/2018/09/07/richard-sackler-member-of-family-behind-oxycontin-was-granted-patent-for-addiction-treatment/.

[30] "Pharma Lobbying Held Deep Influence over Opioid Policies." *Center for Public Integrity*, September 18, 2016. https://publicintegrity.org/politics/state-politics/pharma-lobbying-held-deep-influence-over-opioid-policies/.

[31] Knauth, Dietrich. "Purdue Pharma, Sacklers Reach $7.4 Billion National Opioid Settlement." *Reuters*, January 23, 2025. https://www.reuters.com/business/healthcare-pharmaceuticals/purdue-pharma-sacklers-reach-74-bln-national-opioid-settlement-2025-01-23/

[32] Pytell, Jarratt D., and Darius A. Rastegar. "Who Leaves Early? Factors Associated With Against Medical Advice Discharge During Alcohol Withdrawal Treatment." *Journal of Addiction Medicine* 12, no. 6 (November 2018): 447-52. doi: 10.1097/adm.0000000000000430.

[33] Kelly, John F. "The New Science on Addiction Recovery." *Recovery Research Institute*, Massachusetts General Hospital, 2020. https://www.recoveryanswers.org/research-post/the-new-science-on-addiction-recovery/.

[34] "Treatment and Recovery." *National Institute on Drug Abuse*, July 6, 2020. https://nida.nih.gov/publications/drugs-brains-behavior-science-addiction/treatment-recovery.

[35] Grisel, Judith. *Never Enough: The Neuroscience and Experience of Addiction*. New York: Doubleday, 2019.

[36] "Neuroscience: The Brain in Addiction and Recovery." *National Institute on Alcohol Abuse and Alcoholism*, last modified May 8, 2025. https://www.niaaa.nih.gov/health-professionals-communities/core-resource-on-alcohol/neuroscience-brain-addiction-and-recovery.

[37] Haskell, Brittany. "Identification and Evidence-Based Treatment of Post-Acute Withdrawal Syndrome." *The Journal for Nurse Practitioners* 18, no. 3 (2022): 272-275. doi: 10.1016/j.nurpra.2021.12.021.

[38] Lewis, M. (2015). *The Biology of Desire.*

[39] Carroll, Kathleen M. "Cognitive Behavioral Interventions for Alcohol and Drug Use Disorders." *Psychiatric Clinics of North America* 40, no. 3 (2017): 511-525. doi: 10.1016/j.psc.2017.04.003.

[40] Carroll, Kathleen M., Brian D. Kiluk, Nancy M. Nich, et al. "Computer-Assisted Delivery of Cognitive-Behavioral Therapy: Efficacy and Durability of CBT4CBT Among Cocaine-Dependent Individuals Maintained on Methadone." *American Journal of Psychiatry* 171, no. 4 (2014): 436-444. doi: 10.1176/appi.ajp.2013.13070987.

[41] Prendergast, Michael, Debra Podus, Steve Finney, Alison Greenwell, and S. Roll. "Contingency Management for Treatment of Substance Use Disorders: A Meta-Analysis." *Addiction* 101, no. 11 (2006): 1546-1560. doi: 10.1111/j.1360-0443.2006.01581.x.

[42] Volkow, Nora D., and A. Thomas McLellan. "Medication-Assisted Thera-

Bibliography

pies—Tackling the Opioid-Overdose Epidemic." *New England Journal of Medicine* 370, no. 22 (2014): 2063-2066. doi: 10.1056/NEJMp1402780.

[43] Bowen, Sarah, Katie Witkiewitz, Neha Hsu, and G. Alan Marlatt. "Mindfulness-Based Relapse Prevention for Substance Use Disorders: A Pilot Efficacy Trial." *Substance Abuse* 29, no. 4 (2008): 295-305. doi: 10.1080/08897070802257967.

[44] Substance Abuse and Mental Health Services Administration. *National Survey of Substance Abuse Treatment Services (N-SSATS): 2020.* Rockville, MD: SAMHSA, 2021. https://www.samhsa.gov/data/sites/default/files/reports/rpt35313/2020_NSSATS_FINAL.pdf.

[45] Kelly, John F., and Keith Humphreys. "Alcoholics Anonymous and 12-Step Facilitation Treatments for Alcohol Use Disorder." *Cochrane Database of Systematic Reviews* 3, no. CD012880 (2020). doi: 10.1002/14651858.CD012880.pub2/full.

[46] Mehta, Dinesh D., et al. "A Systematic Review and Meta-Analysis of Neuromodulation Therapies for Substance Use Disorders." *Neuropsychopharmacology* 48, no. 1 (2023): 1-12. doi: 10.1038/s41386-023-01776-0.

[47] Huang, Q., et al. "Virtual Reality-Based Cue Exposure Therapy Reduces Psychological Craving in Methamphetamine Use Disorder." *Translational Psychiatry* 15, no. 1 (2025): Article 123. doi: 10.1038/s41398-025-03553-7.

[48] Sachdeva, Nitin, et al. "Readmissions After Alcohol Detoxification: A Nationwide Analysis." *Alcohol and Alcoholism* 53, no. 4 (2018): 448-454. doi: 10.1093/alcalc/agy027.

[49] Lewis, David. "The 30-Day Myth." *Los Angeles Times*, November 10, 2008. https://www.latimes.com/archives/la-xpm-2008-nov-10-he-addiction10-story.html.

[50] Staples, John, et al. "Leaving Hospital Early Linked With Higher Drug Overdose Risk." *Medscape*, October 1, 2024. https://www.medscape.com/viewarticle/leaving-hospital-early-linked-higher-drug-overdose-risk-2024a1000hu3.

[51] Substance Abuse and Mental Health Services Administration (SAMHSA). *Treatment Episode Data Set (TEDS) 2022: Discharges from Substance Use Treatment Services,* 2022. https://www.samhsa.gov/data/sites/default/files/reports/rpt53160/2022-teds-annual-report.pdf.

[52] Rodríguez, M. N., et al. "Differences by Gender, PTSD Status, and Chronic Pain in Trauma Exposure Among Individuals Receiving Medication for Opioid Use Disorder." *Substance Abuse: Research and Treatment*, 2024. doi: 10.1177/13011412221122222.

[53] Broekhof, R., H.M. Nordahl, Lars Tanum, and S. G. Selvik. "Adverse Childhood Experiences and Their Association with Substance Use Disorders in Adulthood: A General Population Study (Young-HUNT)." *Addictive Behaviors Reports* 17 (2023): 100488. doi:10.1016/j.abrep.2023.100488.

[54] Maté, G. (2008). *In the Realm of Hungry Ghosts.*

[55] Newman, Katelyn. "Treating the Trauma Behind Addiction." *U.S. News &*

Bibliography

World Report, May 2019. https://www.usnews.com/news/healthiest-commu
nities/articles/2019-05-10/joe-polish-treat-the-trauma-behind-addiction.

[56] Samples, Hillary, Arthur Robin Williams, Stephen Crystal, and Mark
Olfson. "Psychosocial and Behavioral Therapy in Conjunction with
Medication for Opioid Use Disorder: Patterns, Predictors, and Association
with Buprenorphine Treatment Outcomes." *Journal of Substance Abuse Treatment* 139 (2022): 108774. doi: 10.101.

[57] Amen, Daniel G. *Change Your Brain, Change Your Life.* Amen Clinics, 2013.

[58] *Substance Use Disorder Treatment and Family Therapy.* Rockville, MD: Substance
Abuse and Mental Health Services Administration, 2020.

[59] National Council on Alcoholism and Drug Dependence. "Family Disease."
NCADD. Accessed October 27, 2025. https://ncadd.us/family-friends/
there-is-help/family-disease.

[60] Esteban, Jessica, Cristian Suárez-Relinque, and Teresa I. Jiménez. "Effects
of Family Therapy for Substance Abuse: A Systematic Review of Recent
Research." *Family Process* (2022).

[61] "Substance Abuse Statistics for Native Americans." *American Addiction
Centers*, May 2, 2025. https://americanaddictioncenters.org/rehab-guide/
addiction-statistics-demographics/native-americans.

[62] Center for Behavioral Health Statistics and Quality. "2017 National
Survey on Drug Use and Health: Detailed Tables." (2018): 1-2871.

[63] Jezewski, Mary Ann, and Kathryn M. Sotnik. "Addressing Diverse Populations in Intensive Outpatient and Aftercare Programs: Chapter 10." *Diversity
and Addiction: Helping People from Diverse Cultures*, 149-69. Champaign, IL:
Research Press, 2005.

[64] Brave Heart, Maria Yellow Horse. "The Historical Trauma Response
Among Natives and Its Relationship with Substance Abuse: A Lakota Illus-
tration." *Journal of Psychoactive Drugs* 35, no. 1 (2003): 7-13. doi:
10.1080/02791072.2003.10399988.

[65] Williams, David R., and Selina A. Mohammed. "Racism and Health
Inequities: The Role of Structural Racism." *Public Health Reports* 125, no. 1
(2010): 37-48.

[66] Guerrero, Erick, Sara A. Marsh, and Louise K. Lambert. "Understanding
Barriers to Specialty Substance Abuse Treatment among Latinos." *Journal
of Substance Abuse Treatment* 87 (2018): 1-8.

[67] Budge, Stephanie L., et al. "Exploring the Experiences of LGBTQ+ Individuals in Substance Use Treatment Services: A Qualitative Study."
Substance Abuse Treatment, Prevention, and Policy 18 (2023): 1-11.

[68] Nasta, Luke, and Patricia Strach. "What Drives Staffing Levels for
Substance-Use Disorder (SUD) Services in New York State?" *The Rockefeller
Institute of Government*, Report No. 41 (2021).

[69] Proctor, Sherry L. "The Continuing Care Model of Substance Use Treatment." *Journal of Substance Abuse Treatment* 46, no. 2 (2014): 120-130.

[70] Williams, Alex M., and Susan L. Mackler. "Insurance Barriers to Addic-

tion Treatment: The Role of Prior-Authorization and Service-Limits in Substance Use Disorder Care." *Journal of Substance Abuse Treatment* 148 (2024): 108964. doi:10.1016/j.jsat.2023.108964.

[71] Reilly, Cynthia, and Samantha Arsenault. "Insurance Coverage for Substance Use Disorder Treatment Impedes Care." *The Pew Charitable Trusts*, March 29, 2017.

[72] Dispenza, Joe. *Breaking the Habit of Being Yourself: How to Lose Your Mind and Create a New One.* Carlsbad, CA: Hay House, 2012.

[73] Miller, Jessica. "Social Media Addiction Statistics - Risks, Warnings & Safety (2025)." *AddictionHelp.com*, last updated October 19, 2025. https://www.addictionhelp.com/social-media-addiction/statistics/.

[74] Cape, G. S. "Addiction, Stigma and Movies." *Acta Psychiatrica Scandinavica* 107, no. 3 (February 7, 2003): 163-69. https://doi.org/10.1034/j.1600-0447.2003.00075.x.

[75] Roberts, Donald F., Lisa Henriksen, and Peter G. Christianson. *Substance Use in Popular Movies and Music.* Washington, DC: U.S. Department of Justice, Office of Justice Programs, April 1999.

[76] Kelly, John F., and C. M. Westerhoff. "Does It Matter How We Refer to Individuals with Substance-Related Conditions? A Randomised Study of Two Commonly Used Terms." *International Journal of Drug Policy* 21, no. 3 (2010): 202-207. doi: 10.1016/j.drugpo.2009.10.010.

[77] Sinha, Rajita. "Stress and Substance Use Disorders: Risk, Relapse, and Treatment Implications." *Psychosocial Intervention* 33, no. 1 (2024): 25-35. doi: 10.5093/pi2024a5.

[78] Teplin, Linda A., et al. "Incarceration-Related Exposure and Overdose Risk: Formerly Incarcerated Persons Are Up to 40 Times More Likely to Die of an Opioid Overdose than the General Population." *Healthy People 2030 Literature Summaries – Incarceration* (U.S. Office of Disease Prevention and Health Promotion), last modified 2024. https://odphp.health.gov/healthypeople/priority-areas/social-determinants-health/literature-summaries/incarceration.

[79] Maté, G. (2008). *In the Realm of Hungry Ghosts.*

[80] Rêgo, Ximene, Maria João Oliveira, Catarina Lameira, and Olga S. Cruz. "20 Years of Portuguese Drug Policy – Developments, Challenges and the Quest for Human Rights." *Substance Abuse Treatment, Prevention, and Policy* 16 (2021): 59. doi: 10.1186/s13011-021-00394-7.

[81] Collins, Susan E., Heather S. Lonczak, and Seema L. Clifasefi. "Seattle's Law Enforcement Assisted Diversion (Lead): Program Effects on Recidivism Outcomes." *Evaluation and Program Planning* 64 (October 2017): 49-56. doi: 10.1016/j.evalprogplan.2017.05.008.

[82] Lurigio, Arthur J. "The First 20 Years of Drug Treatment Courts: A Brief Description of Their History and Impact." *Federal Probation* 72, no. 1 (2008): 8-12.

[83] Office of National Drug Control Policy. "Drug Courts: A Smart Approach

Bibliography

to Criminal Justice." Washington, DC: White House, 2015. https://obamawhitehouse.archives.gov/ondcp/ondcp-fact-sheets/drug-courts-smart-approach-to-criminal-justice.

[84] National Association of State Alcohol and Drug Abuse Directors (NASADAD). *State Regulation of Substance Use Disorder Programs and Counselors.* Washington, DC: NASADAD, July 2013.

[85] Clingan, S. E. "Patient Brokering in For-Profit Substance Use Disorder Treatment Facilities." *BMC Health Services Research* 23 (2023): 569. doi: 10.1186/s12913-023-10217-z.

[86] Hudetz, Mary, and Hannah Bassett. "Dozens Died in Sober Living Homes as Arizona Fumbled Fraud Crackdown." *ProPublica/Arizona Center for Investigative Reporting,* January 27, 2025.

[87] Dispenza, J. (2012). *Breaking the Habit of Being Yourself.*

[88] Lehrer, Paul M., Karenjot Kaur, Agratta Sharma, Khushbu Shah, Robert Huseby, Jay Bhavsar, and Yingting Zhang. "Heart Rate Variability Biofeedback Improves Emotional and Physical Health and Performance: A Systematic Review and Meta-Analysis." *Applied Psychophysiology and Biofeedback* 45, no. 2 (2020): 109-129. doi: 10.1007/s10484-020-09466-z.

About the Author

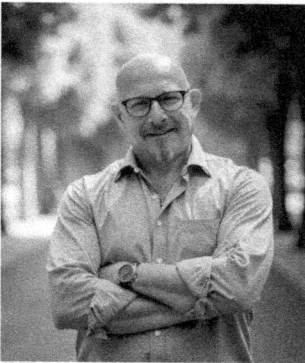

Jimmie Applegate is a transformational consultant and author with over 30 years of experience in organizational and personal change. As a certified Neuro-ChangeSolutions Consultant and HeartMath practitioner, Applegate is also a certified Peer and Recovery Support Specialist, US Air Force veteran, dedicated husband and father of four.

The owner and Administrative Director of Beacon Treatment Center, Applegate guides people in recovery from addiction to develop the skills, mindset and resilience needed for lasting transformation. *Addicted to Failure: Why the Rehab System Doesn't Work and What Must Change* is his first book.

For more information about Jimmie Applegate and his work, scan the QR code below:

About the Publisher

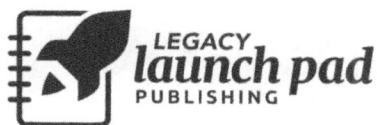

Legacy Launch Pad is a boutique publishing company that works with entrepreneurs from all over the world. For more information about Legacy Launch Pad Publishing, go to: www.legacylaunchpadpub.com.

www.ingramcontent.com/pod-product-compliance
Lightning Source LLC
Chambersburg PA
CBHW022055020426
42335CB00012B/693